Embryology - Theory and Practice

Edited by Bin Wu and Huai L. Feng

Published in London, United Kingdom

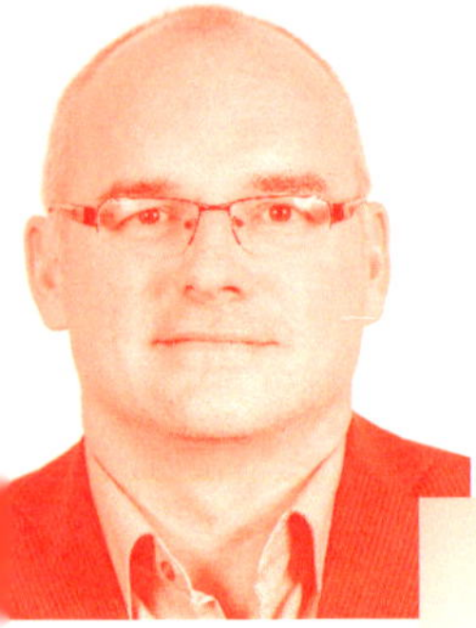
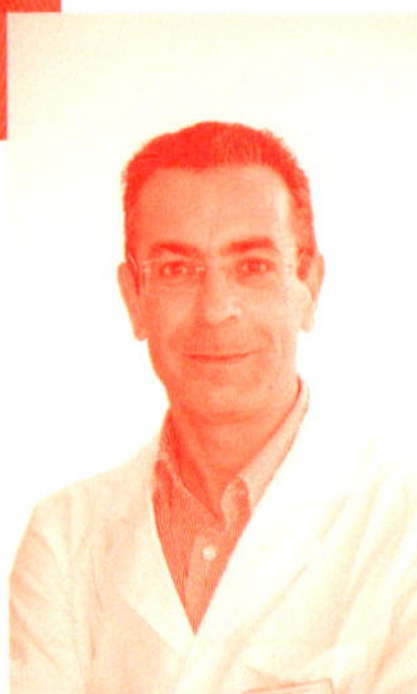
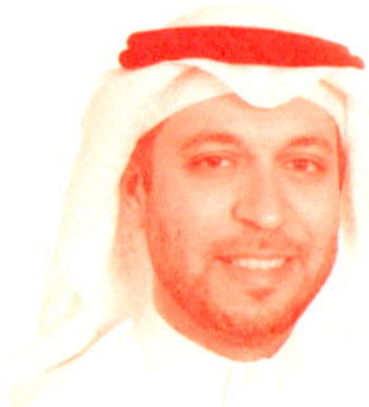
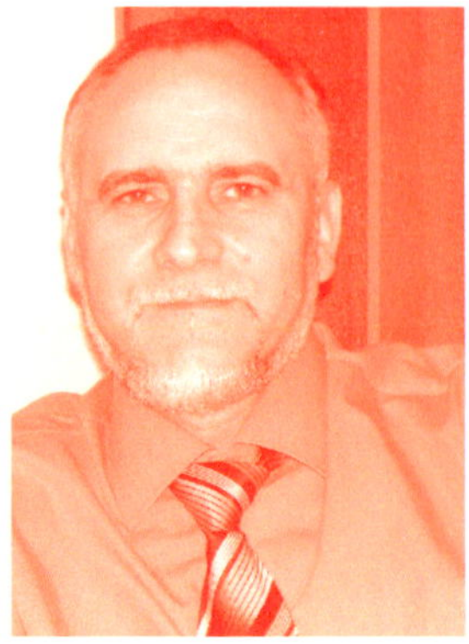
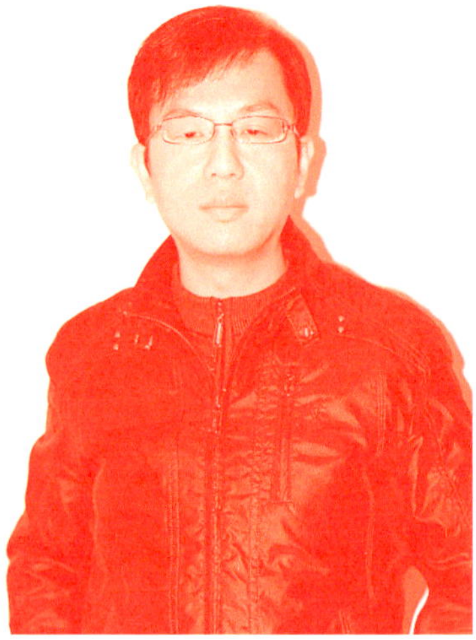
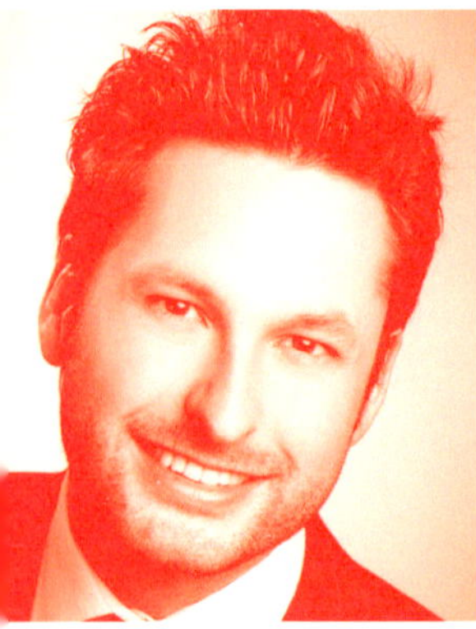
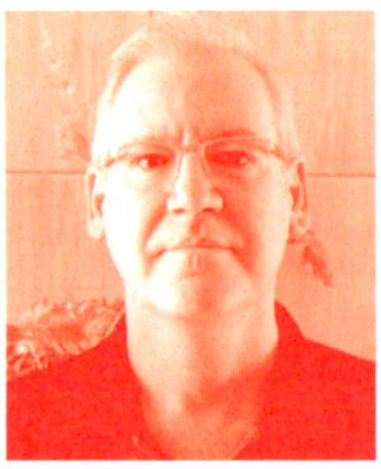

IntechOpen

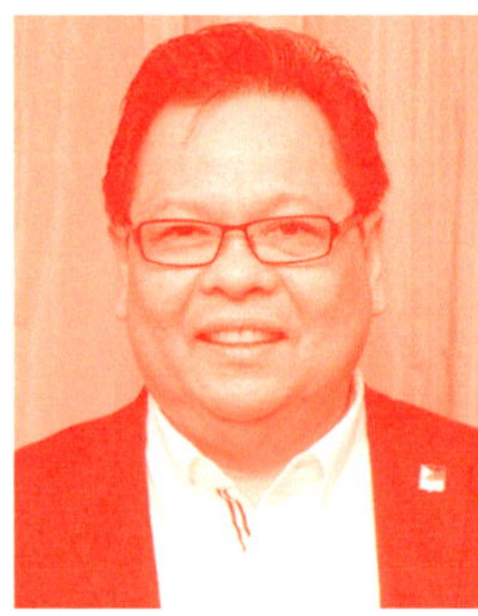
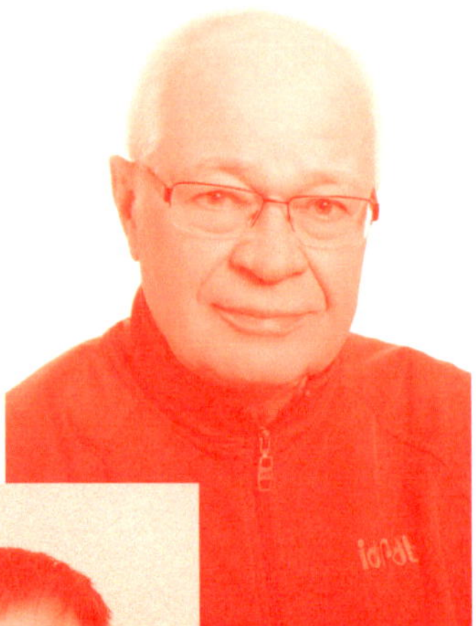
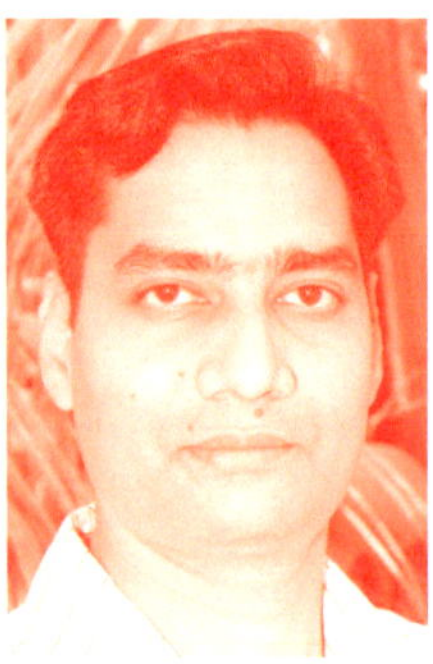
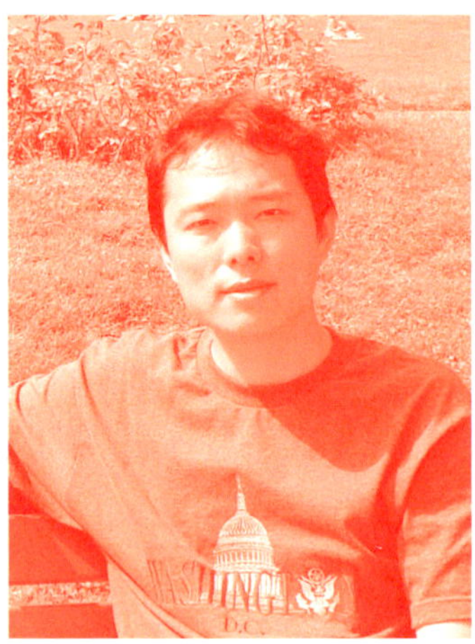
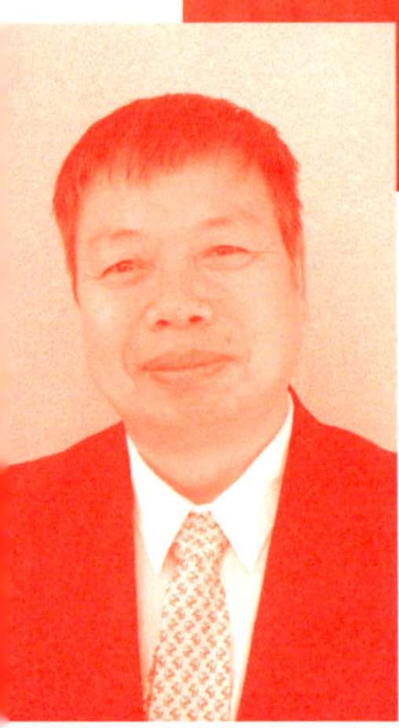
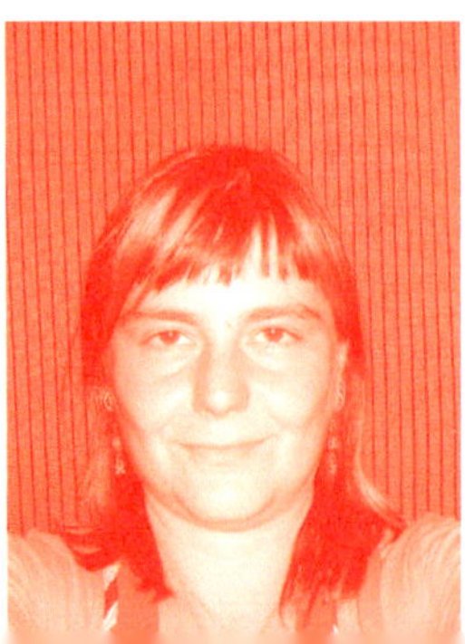

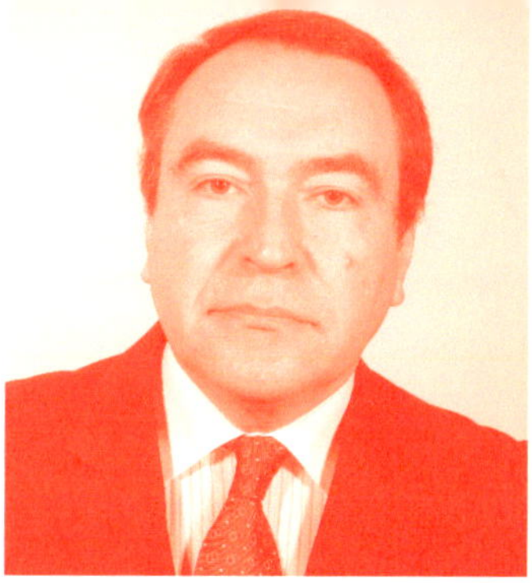
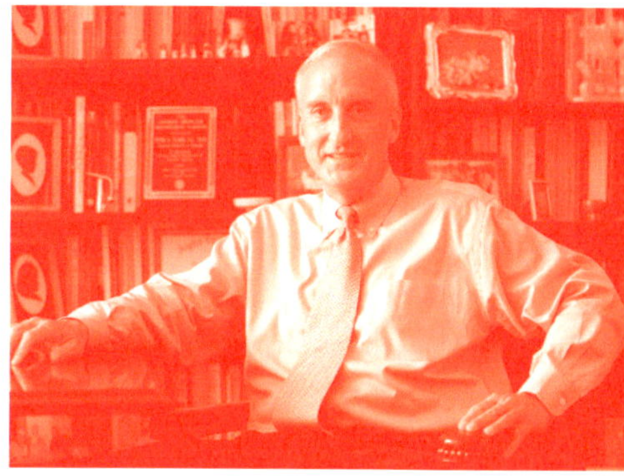
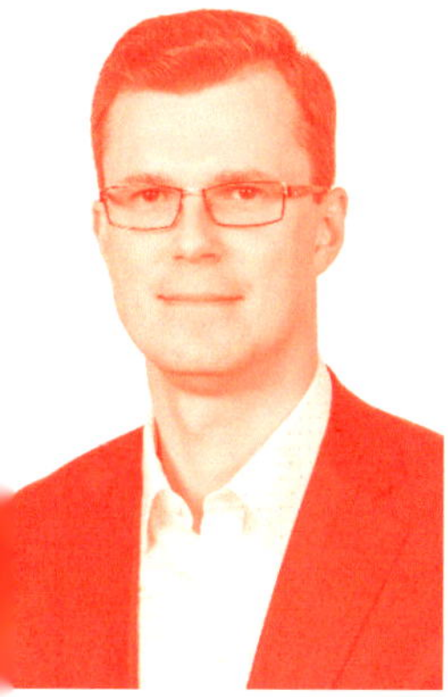
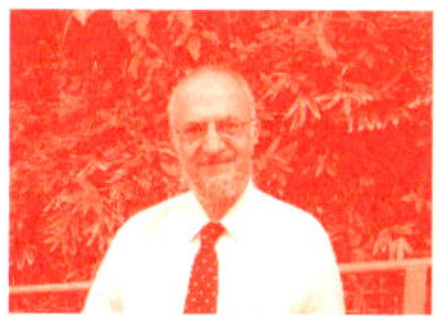
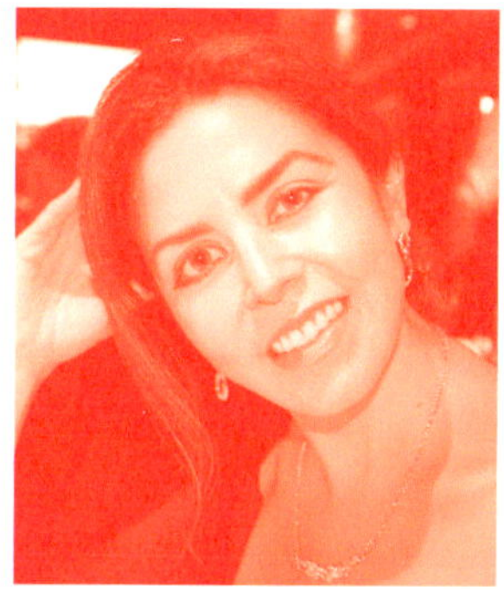

Supporting open minds since 2005

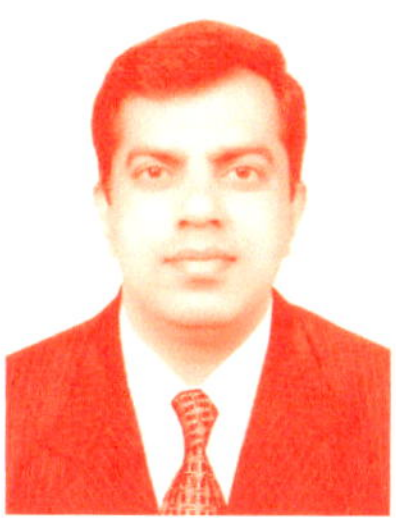
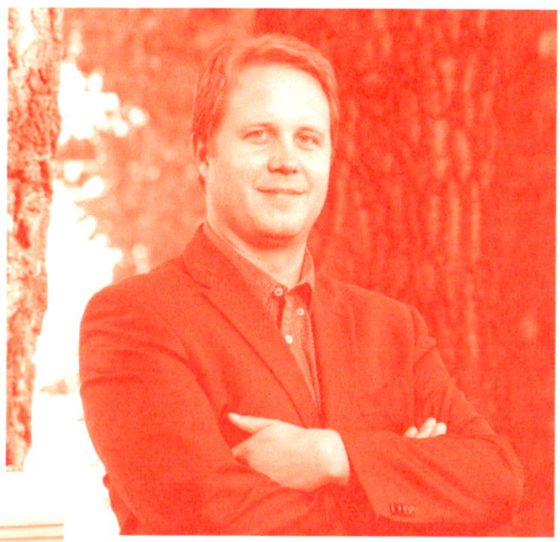
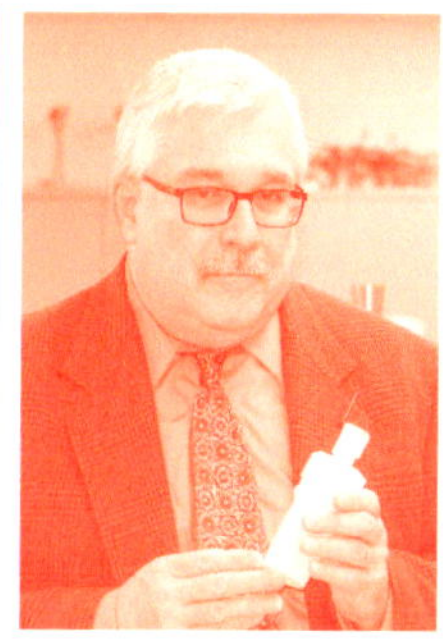
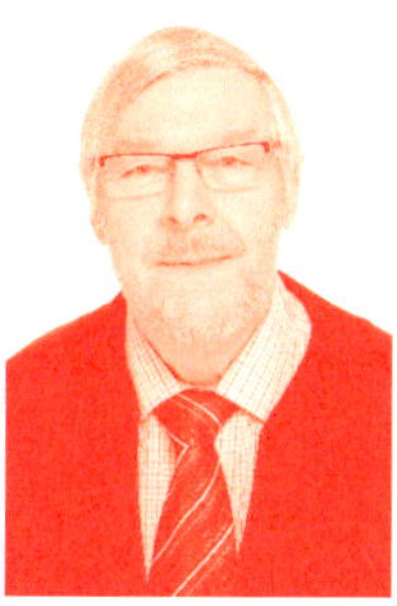
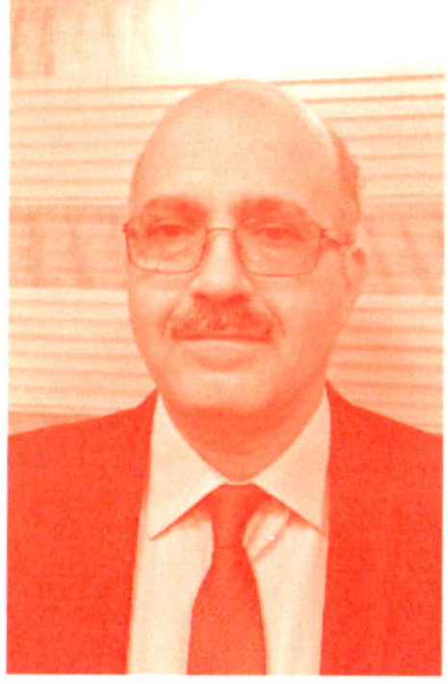
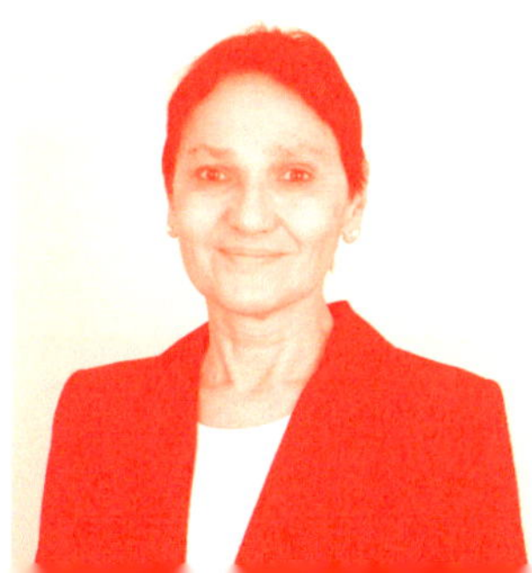
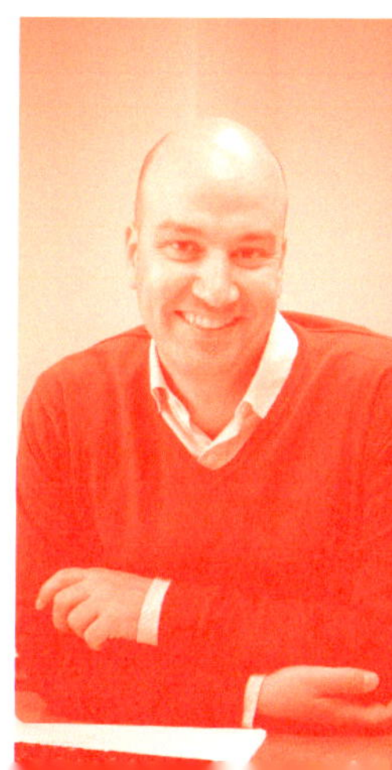

Embryology - Theory and Practice
http://dx.doi.org/10.5772/intechopen.73724
Edited by Bin Wu and Huai L. Feng

Contributors
Iavor K. Vladimirov, Desislava Tacheva, Vladislav Dobrinov, Goran Mitulović, Tanja Panić-Janković, Borut Kovačič, Nina Hojnik, Hilma Putri Lubis, Binarwan Halim, Fernando Moreira Da Silva, Loide Valadão, Helena Moreira Da Silva, Bin Wu, Linda Wu, Jinzhou Qin, Dikai Zhang, Minqi Zhang, Suzhen Lu, Timothy Gelety, Jennifer Howell, Xiaolin La, Jing Zhao, Zhihui Wang, Rong Li, Fen-Ting Liu

First published in London, United Kingdom, 2019 by IntechOpen
IntechOpen is the global imprint of INTECHOPEN LIMITED, registered in England and Wales, registration number: 11086078, The Shard, 25th floor, 32 London Bridge Street
London, SE19SG - United Kingdom
Printed in Croatia

British Library Cataloguing-in-Publication Data
A catalogue record for this book is available from the British Library

Additional hard and PDF copies can be obtained from orders@intechopen.com

Embryology - Theory and Practice
Edited by Bin Wu and Huai L. Feng
p. cm.
Print ISBN 978-1-78985-305-6
Online ISBN 978-1-78985-306-3
eBook (PDF) ISBN 978-1-78985-639-2

For EU product safety concerns:
IN TECH d.o.o., Prolaz Marije Krucifikse Kozulić 3, 51000 Rijeka, Croatia, info@intechopen.com or visit our website at intechopen.com.

Meet the editors

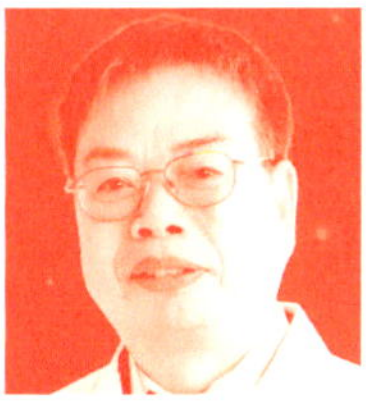

Bin Wu, PhD, HCLD, is currently a scientific laboratory director at the Arizona Center for Reproductive Endocrinology and Infertility, USA. He received his training in genetics and reproductive biology at the Northwest Agricultural University in China and Cornell University, New York, and his postdoctor training at the University of Guelph, Canada. He was then promoted to professor at the Northwest Agricultural University. Dr. Wu has membership of many professional associations, including the American Society for Reproductive Medicine, the International Embryo Transfer Society, and has also obtained significant research awards from these professional associations. The American College of Embryology recognized Dr. Wu's excellence in the practice of reproductive embryology in July 2014.

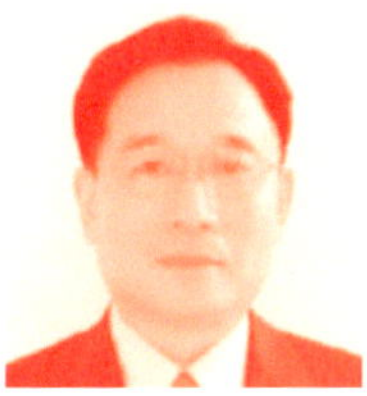

Dr. Feng is the Director of Infertility/In Vitro Fertilization Laboratories at the New York Presbyterian Health System, Affiliated Weill Medical College of Cornell University. He has served as professor, guest, and honorary professor at a number of other universities and institutions. Dr. Feng is an active member of many academic societies, such as ASRM, ASA, and AAAS, and has served as an editor and ad hoc reviewer for several reproduction-related journals, such as *Human Reproduction Update*, *Human Reproduction*, and *Fertility and Sterility*. He has held over 25 research grants, published more than 200 research papers in peer-reviewed scientific journals, and edited four books as editor-in-chief and co-chief. He has also received more than 30 prizes and awards from professional committees and international organizations. Dr. Feng has presented over 100 invited lectures at international and domestic conferences and workshops. He has been selected as one of the leading scientists of the World 2005 IBC, Cambridge, UK, and as an outstanding inspector from CAP in 2006. He was also the recipient of the 2014 Star Award from the American Society for Reproductive Medicine (ASRM).

Contents

Preface

Since early in the last century, many studies have focused on revealing the mechanism of fertilization and embryo formation and development, which form a branch discipline of biology science, known as embryology. Embryology is a vast discipline concerned with the study of embryogenesis and is the branch of biology that studies the prenatal development of gametes, fertilization, and development of embryos and fetuses. Additionally, embryology encompasses the study of congenital disorders that occur before birth, known as teratology. Findings in embryology have helped in the understanding of congenital abnormalities and developing assisted reproduction procedures.

To date, embryology has been enriched and developed greatly in terms of its contents and forms. It not only includes oogenesis, spermiogenesis, embryogenesis, implantation, and fetal formation mechanisms, but also involves pharmacology, basic scientific research, and regenerative medicine. Although this subject has been studied for more than a century, it is still a pioneering field with many alternative aspects, such as embryonic stem cells, somatic cell cloning, and many novel discoveries appearing continuously. In particular, novel embryo biotechnologies have initiated a new era in the fields of medical science and agriculture because of their enormous biomedical and commercial potential. Thus, the purpose of this book is to update and review newly developed theories and technologies in assisted reproductive technologies (ARTs) and to provide clinical practice examples so that readers, especially embryologists and physicians involved in human IVF programs, may acquire new and usable information as well as key practice techniques.

This book updates new technologies, theories, and methods in early embryogenesis from ovarian stimulation to final ART outcomes. Areas covered include details of background proteins in human chorionic gonadotropin pharmaceutical formulations of different origins; clinical application of *in vitro* maturation of oocytes; oocyte fertilization failure and oocyte activation, both physiological and clinical aspects; human blastocyst formation and development; bovine embryonic development to implantation; the role of neuroendocrines in embryo implantation; and the present and future of embryo cryopreservation and effect of ART on newborn babies. Thus, this book will provide some important information for readers, especially embryologists and physicians for human IVF programs to improve their appreciation of ART.

Bin Wu, PhD, HCLD (ABB)
Arizona Center for Reproductive Endocrinology and Infertility,
Tucson, Arizona, USA

Huai L. Feng, PhD, HCLD, ELD
Department of Obstetrics and Gynecology,
New York Hospital Queens,
Weill Medical College,
Cornell University,
New York, USA

Section 1

Introduction

Chapter 1

Introductory Chapter: New Theory and Technology in Early Clinical Embryogenesis

Bin Wu

1. Introduction

Embryology has a long history. Since early last century, many studies focused on revealing the mechanism of the fertilization and embryo formation and development, which formed a branch discipline of biology science, that is, embryology. Embryology is a vast discipline concerned with the study of embryogenesis, and it is the branch of biology that studies the prenatal development of gametes, fertilization, and development of embryos and fetuses. Additionally, embryology encompasses the study of congenital disorders that occur before birth, known as teratology [1, 2]. Findings in embryology have helped in the understanding of congenital abnormalities and developing assisted reproduction procedures.

To date, embryology has been enriched and developed greatly in the terms of its contents and forms. It not only includes oogenesis, spermiogenesis, embryogenesis, implantation, and fetal formation mechanism, but also involves pharmacology, basic scientific research, and regenerative medicine. Although this subject has been studied for more than a century, it is still a pioneering field with many alternative aspects such as embryonic stem cell, somatic cell cloning, and many novel discoveries that appear continuously. Particularly, some novel embryo biotechnologies have initiated a new era in the fields of medical science and agriculture owing to their enormous biomedical and commercial potential.

In the last four decades, the assisted reproductive technology (ART) has created some new observations and novel discoveries in the early stage of embryogenesis, especially in preimplantation from gametogenesis to blastocyst embryo formation in vitro (**Figure 1**).

Thus, this book contains some novel discoveries and theories on the embryology field in last the decade.

The key technique of the assisted reproductive technology is in vitro fertilization (IVF). Since this technique's creation, the current developed methods have been widely used for the treatment of infertile couples to make them realize their dream to

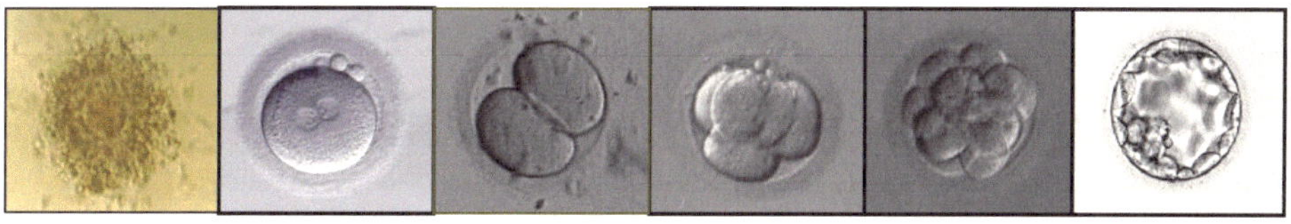

Figure 1.
Human embryogenesis from oocyte to blastocyst stage during preimplantation.

have a baby. Currently, these technologies mainly contain in vitro fertilization (IVF) and its related procedures—intracytoplasmic sperm injection (ICSI), frozen embryo transfer (FET), and preimplantation genetic testing (PGT) for aneuploidies (PGT-A, previously known as PGS), for monogenic/single-gene defects (PGT-M, previously known as PGD), and for chromosomal structural rearrangements (PGT-SR, previously known as PGD Screen (PGS)). [Note: New PGT nomenclature announced by the International Committee Monitoring Assisted Reproductive Technologies (ICMART) in collaboration with the American Society for Reproductive Medicine (ASRM), European Society of Human Reproduction and Embryology (ESHRE), and other professional medical societies, 2018] [3]. So far, more than 10 million IVF/ICSI and frozen embryo transfer babies have been born throughout the world. This technique indeed gives many infertile families to bring happy life. Although this technology has been widely used in human infertile treatment and animal industry, it also faces some problems which need to be resolved, such as low embryo development rate, low pregnant rate, as well as birth baby health. Thus, some continuous improvements on this technology have been happening now. Firstly, in order to obtain good quality eggs, ovarian stimulation needs to use some high-quality medicines such as gonadotropins, including human chorionic gonadotropin (hCG), which is the most important reproductive hormone for embryogenesis and embryo development and implantation in the uterus [4–6]. Thus, we should concern the total hCG protein content varied from batch to batch and a large number of contaminant urinary proteins identified in all analyzed samples except for the recombinant product. The good quality hCG application will improve embryo quality and pregnant rate.

In vitro maturation (IVM) is a technique used to induce in vitro maturation of immature oocytes collected from ovarian follicles without any medication stimulation. In a routine IVF practice, several kinds of gonadotropins are used to produce more mature eggs for fertilization every egg retrieval cycle. This procedure is widely used in most of the IVF centers, but the application of these drugs obviously increases fertility treatment cost, and patients also suffer many times from drug injections. In IVF practice, another pathway is oocyte in vitro maturation; that is, without ovarian stimulation, immature oocytes are retrieved from ovary and conducted for maturation under the laboratory condition for about 24 h in vitro, subsequent for normal insemination. Currently this technology has achieved some success, but it needs to be further improved to obtain a higher pregnant rate. Thus, IVM application significantly reduces IVF cost, patient emotional address and side effects, and frequent hospital visits [7].

At beginning, IVM technique was designed as an alternative to conventional IVF for minimizing the risk of the ovarian hyperstimulation syndrome (OHSS) in patients with the polycystic ovarian syndrome (PCOS). As an effective treatment method, IVM can be used to treat patients with polycystic ovary syndrome, ovarian hyperresponsiveness, and hyporesponsiveness, as well as to preserve the fertility of cancer patients [8]. This technology has been used worldwide for the birth of thousands of healthy babies. The improvement in clinical IVM technology mainly focuses on the IVM medium and the optimization of the culture environment and operation process. Recently many research groups have started to combine clinical application of IVM with a natural cycle or mild stimulation in IVF practice, especially for PCOS and age women. In particular, the combination of mild stimulation IVF with IVM is not only expected to become a viable alternative to current standard treatments, but may also become a potential option of first-line treatment.

After obtaining MII oocytes, a key technique is oocyte insemination with sperm including in vitro fertilization and intracytoplasmic sperm injection in order to obtain normal fertilized egg, that is, zygote. ICSI technique has greatly improved normal IVF fertilization failure and increased oocyte fertilization rate and solved severe male infertility problem [9], which has made many infertile males realize their dream to have children in their family. However, some fertilization failures still appear on good quality oocytes. Thus, oocyte activation is also very important for fertilization. The incidence and etiology of total fertilization failure after ICSI have led embryologists to search new activation studies including physiology of oocyte activation, electrical properties of gametes' membranes, and ion currents. It is very important that calcium oscillation is an essential process during oocyte activation. Many researches have shown that oocyte activation is triggered by sperm factor [10, 11]. Artificial oocyte activation (AOA) also imitates sperm factor function to stimulate oocyte activation for successful fertilization. Artificial activation can be induced by the use of electrical, mechanical, or chemical stimuli to elevate intracellular concentrations of calcium ions [12]. Thus, discussion on the effect of different AOA methods on the success and safety will help embryologists to improve fertilization rate and reduce fertilization failure accident.

As shown in **Figure 1**, after fertilization, the embryo experiences a series of events including the formation of the maternal and paternal pronuclei (2PN) on day 1 and cleavage stage on day 1.5 to day 3, reaching the morula (compaction) on day 4 and the blastocyst on day 5, until it arrives at the uterus, where it "hatches" from the zona pellucida to implant into the endometrium. During this period, some important findings are obtained from many IVF practices. Thus, understanding human and animal blastocyst formation and development and their physiology, morphology, and gene expression of blastocyst will help us to reveal the reason for high rate of embryo implantation failure. All these processes for embryonic development need neuroendocrine regulation. Neuroendocrine, an integration of the nervous system and endocrine system as its name implies, plays a critical role in the reproductive system. However, less progress has been made in the particular effects of neuroendocrine on embryo implantation. Despite these barriers, significant knowledge has been gained through recent studies and shows that neuroendocrine is tightly involved in embryo implantation. Therefore, the current state of knowledge about the impaction of neuroendocrine on embryo implantation could make us consider a potential strategy to get higher pregnancy rate after in vitro fertilization and embryo transfer (IVF-ET) in order to decrease recurrent implantation failure (RIF) possibility through modulating the neuroendocrine systems [13, 14].Another important branch in IVF practice is embryo cryopreservation. Embryo freezing technologies have widely been developed and used in human IVF practice and animal industry [15, 16]. In the last decade, the cryopreservation of reproductive cells including stem cells, embryos, gametes, tissues, and organs has become a routine work in many IVF centers and animal industry [17]. As the embryo freezing number increases, some new techniques for cryopreservation have been developed, especially oocyte and embryo vitrification, which have greatly improved oocyte and embryo survival rate after thawing or warming [16]. It is very interesting that a new "Theory About the Embryo-Cryo Treatment" has been formed. It should be considered that the method of cryopreservation is not only a technology for storing embryos but also a method of embryo treatment that can potentially improve the success rates in infertile couples. This theory believes that freezing and thawing process could activate endogenous survival and repair mechanisms in preimplantation embryos. We think that the embryonic thawing process induces low levels of stress, which results in hormesis and could repair mitochondrial damage and protein misfolding. Thus, this theory may explain the higher success rate of frozen-thawing embryo transfer than fresh embryo transfer for age women and the higher miscarriage case. Thus, the "treatment" effect of freezing an embryo may explain the higher success rates than fresh embryo transfer. The analysis of facts and suggestions should enable researchers to rethink the position of cryobiology in reproductive medicine.

During the last couple of decades, the assisted reproductive technologies have become one of the fastest developing branches of medicine. Assisted reproductive technology has been widely used for the treatment of infertile couples to realize their dream to have a baby. However, many people are worried about ART baby health outcome. Although many reviews of ART effect on birth babies have been reported, it is very difficult to find a system data about ART outcome on sex ratio and frozen embryo transfer. Our study provides some detailed data about the effect of ART on human birth babies by two country IVF center data. The result showed that ART patient age is significantly older than normal delivered women; the gestation of fresh and frozen embryo transfer has the same as normal deliver baby gestation days, but multi-baby birth women have shorter gestation days; there is no significant difference on early birth between fresh embryo transfer single babies and normal delivered babies, but multi-babies have a higher early birth rate, and frozen embryo transfer has lower early birth rate; there is no significant difference between male and female babies although fresh embryo transfer looks like more male babies and frozen embryo transfer has more female babies; there is no significant difference on the baby weight between ART singleton babies and normal delivered babies, but male baby weight is more than female babies, and multi-baby birth weights have significant lower singletons, while frozen embryo transfer babies have significant heavier birth weight than fresh embryo transfer. These results showed that the singleton with ART treatment does not have any significant difference from normal single babies on gestation days, early birth rate, and baby birth weight, but multi-baby birth often has high early birth rate with shorter gestation day and lower birth weight. The frozen embryo transfer may significantly reduce early birth rate. Thus, frozen embryo transfer may be recommended as a very healthy strategy in ART.

In fine, some new technologies, theories, and methods in early embryogenesis from ovarian stimulation to final ART outcome have been developed in the last decade. The systemic understanding of these new knowledge containing some basic theories and technologies will be helpful for animal scientists and human clinical physicians and embryologists to improve their ART outcome.

Author details

Bin Wu
Arizona Center for Reproductive Endocrinology and Infertility, Tucson, AZ, USA

*Address all correspondence to: bwu13@yahoo.com

References

[1] Rogers JM, Kavlock RJ. Developmental toxicology. In: Klaassen CD, editor. Casarett & Doull's Toxicology. 5th ed. New York: McGraw-Hill; 1996. pp. 301-331. ISBN: 0-07-105476-6

[2] Thall Bastow BD, Holmes JL. Teratology and Drug Use During Pregnancy. Medscape. WebMD. 2016. [Retrieved: February 24, 2016]

[3] The Center for Human Reproduction. PGS No More, Long Live PGT-A. 2017. Available from: https://www.centerforhumanreprod.com/fertility/pgs-no-long-live-pgt

[4] Vrekoussis AMT, Zoumakis E, Kalantaridou SN, Jeschke U. The role of HCG in implantation: A mini-review of molecular and clinical evidence. International Journal of Molecular Sciences. 2017;**18**:1305. DOI: 10.3390/ijms18061305. www.mdpi.com/journal/ijms

[5] Tsampalas M, Gridelet V, Berndt S, Foidart J-M, Geenen V, d'Hauterive SP. Human chorionic gonadotropin: A hormone with immunological and angiogenic properties. Journal of Reproductive Immunology. 2010;**85**(1):93-98

[6] Licht P, Losch A, Dittrich R, Neuwinger J, Siebzehnrubl E, Wildt L. Novel insights into human endometrial paracrinology and embryo-maternal communication by intrauterine microdialysis. Human Reproduction Update. 1998;**4**(5):532-538

[7] Chang EM, Song HS, Lee DR, Lee WS, Yoon TK. In vitro maturation of human oocytes: Its role in infertility treatment and new possibilities. Clinical and Experimental Reproductive Medicine. 2014;**41**(2):41-46

[8] Lonergan P, Fair T. Maturation of oocytes in vitro. Annual Review of Animal Biosciences. 2016;**4**:255-268. DOI: 10.1146/annurev-animal-022114-110822

[9] Wu B, Gelety JT, Shi J. Chapter 8: 2012 advances in fertility options of azoospermic men. In: Wu B, editor. Advances in Embryo Transfer. Croatia: InTech publisher; 2012. pp. 115-132

[10] Flaherty SP, Payne D, Matthews CD. Fertilization failures and abnormal fertilization after intracytoplasmic sperm injection. Human Reproduction. 1998;**13**(Suppl. 1):155-164

[11] Liu J, Nagy Z, Joris H, Tournaye H, Smitz J, Camus M, et al. Analysis of 76 total fertilization failure cycles out of 2732 intracytoplasmic sperm injection cycles. Human Reproduction. 1995;**10**(10):2630-2636

[12] Mansour R, Fahmy I, Tawab NA, Kamal A, El-Demery Y, Aboulghar M, et al. Electrical activation of oocytes after intracytoplasmic sperm injection: A controlled randomized study. Fertility and Sterility [Internet]. 2009;**91**(1):133-139. DOI: 10.1016/j.fertnstert.2007.08.017

[13] Margalioth EJ et al. Investigation and treatment of repeated implantation failure following IVF-ET. Human Reproduction. 2006;**21**(12):3036-3043

[14] Ashary N, Tiwari A, Modi D. Embryo implantation: War in times of love. Endocrinology. 2018;**159**(2):1188-1198. DOI: 10.1210/en.2017-03082

[15] Whittingham D, Leibo S, Mazur P. Survival of mouse embryos frozen to −196 and −269°C. Science. 1972;**178**(4059):411-414. DOI: 10.1126/science.178.4059.411

[16] Gosden R. Prospects for oocyte banking and in vitro maturation. Journal of the National Cancer Institute. Monographs. 2005;**2005**(34):60-63. DOI: 10.1093/jncimonographs/lgi007

[17] Woods E, Benson J, Agca Y, Critser J. Fundamental cryobiology of reproductive cells and tissues. Cryobiology. 2004;**48**(2):146-156. DOI: 10.1016/j.cryobiol.2004.03.002

Section 2

Ovarian Stimulation, Ooctye Maturation and Fertilization

Chapter 2

Background Proteins in Human Chorionic Gonadotropin Pharmaceutical Formulations of Different Origins

Tanja Panić-Janković and Goran Mitulović

Abstract

Gonadotropins, including human chorionic gonadotropin (hCG), have been used since and for several decades to treat infertility by ovarian stimulation. hCG is the most important protein for embryogenesis and embryo development and implantation in uterus upon fertilization of oocytes. The hCG used for in-vitro fertilization (IVF) is being extracted from urine of pregnant women, and it does inevitably contains other proteins secreted into urine. The presence of other proteins varies from batch to batch, and it can be significantly high. Due to the fact that many of the proteins identified in these formulations can trigger an allergic reaction, which, in turn, can affect the embryogenesis and prevent embryo implantation, it is very important to check the amount and type of contaminant proteins in pharmaceutical formulations. It was found that the total protein content varied from batch to batch, and a large number of contaminant urinary proteins were identified in all analyzed samples except for the recombinant product.

Keywords: embryogenesis, in-vitro fertilization, human chorionic gonadotropin, proteomics

1. Introduction

Human chorionic gonadotropin (hCG) is one of the most widely studied markers in embryonic development. It is used as an obstetric marker, and it is often regarded as little more than a signal for maternal recognition of pregnancy. Human chorionic gonadotropin is a member of the dimeric glycoprotein hormone family that also includes FSH, LH, and TSH. The members of this hormone family share a common α subunit and have a unique β subunit to each hormone. Additionally, each hormone shows a different level of glycosylation, which determines circulating half-life and receptor binding affinity [1].

The success of embryo implantation upon IVF and embryo transfer depends on various factors related to the embryo quality and patient's endometrial receptivity. Upon implantation, it is important that the embryo reaches the endometrial cavity during the period of time in which the endometrium is receptive. It has been estimated that 50–75% of lost pregnancies are due to the embryo's implantation failure as described by Tsampalas et al. [2]. Many factors are involved in the implantation process, which is very intricate process and the success can be influenced by many factors. The most important regulation of embryogenesis and embryo implantation in uterus is performed by hCG, and studies performed by Licht et al. [3] showed that an intrauterine injection of 500 IU of hCG/mL inhibited the expression of intrauterine insulin-like growth factor-binding protein 1 and the macrophage colony stimulating factor. It was also demonstrated that an intrauterine injection of 500 IU of hCG performed before embryo transfer significantly improved both the implantation and pregnancy rates in IVF/intracytoplasmic sperm injection cycles.

The use of gonadotropin derived from either animal or human tissues was not always without clinical danger (e.g., antibody formation from pregnant mare serum gonadotropin and Creutzfeld-Jacob disease from human pituitary gonadotropin).

The hCG is being extracted from urine of pregnant women (uhCG) for almost three decades, and it is being used for induction of mid-cycle follicular maturation and ovulation in women undergoing an IVF treatment. Originally, hCG in pharmacological preparations was derived only from the urine of pregnant women. However, due to their biological origin, these hCG products show large biological variability and significant batch-to-batch variation. Therefore, recombinant technology has been introduced for the production of recombinant hCG (rhCG) with higher purity and higher batch-to-batch reproducibility and the possibility to control their availability in different doses The availability of different amounts of active substance in recombinant products provides a good starting point to develop personalized therapy for patients depending on their individual hormonal status.

Although a recombinant product is available on the market, urinary preparations of this hormone are still manufactured and are widely used [4–9]. Often, the urinary preparations are associated with problems arising from the fact that the starting material might origin from unknown sources, have poor purity, and lead to large batch-to-batch variations in activity and the amount of other proteins.

Analysis of commercially available, uhCG, was performed earlier [8], and discussions about the possible risks of infection were published [9–15].

We have analyzed several batches of both urinary derived and recombinant hCG formulations and have compared the obtained results in terms of number of identified proteins and their function during the embryogenesis.

2. Materials and methods

2.1 Analyzed hCG: source of the material

Different batches of both uhCG and rhCG were purchased through the pharmacy of the General Hospital of Vienna and by direct purchase from pharmacies in Bosnia-Herzegovina and Serbia. Details on manufacturer and batches analyzed are shown in **Table 1**.

2.2 Proteomics sample preparation

Trypsin for protein digestion was purchased from Promega Inc. (Vienna, Austria). Solvents for HPLC—methanol (MeOH), acetonitrile (AcN), 2,2,2-trifluoroethanol (TFE), formic acid (FA), heptafluorobutyric acid (HFBA), iodoacetamide (IAA), triethyl bicarbonate (TEAB), and dithiothreitol were purchased from Sigma-Aldrich (Vienna, Austria). Digestion of hCG and FSH was performed using the routine approach described in earlier publications [16].

Commercial name and charge number	Dosage	Principal component	Origin	Manufacturer
Pregnyl_M038101	5000 IU/mL	hCG	Urinary-derived	MSD (N.V. organon, NL)
Pregnyl_M011526	5000 IU/mL	hCG	Urinary-derived	MSD (N.V. organon, NL)
Pregnyl_354043	5000 IU/mL	hCG	Urinary-derived	MSD (N.V. organon, NL)
Predalon_117730	5000 IU/mL	hCG	Urinary-derived	MSD (N.V. organon, NL)
Pregnyl_117447	5000 IU/mL	hCG	Urinary-derived	MSD (N.V. organon, NL)
Pregnyl_116935	1500 IU/mL	hCG	Urinary-derived	MSD (N.V. organon, NL)
Pregnyl_M018720	5000 IU/mL	hCG	Urinary-derived	MSD
Chorimon_160432	5000 IU/mL	hCG	Urinary-derived	Institut Biochimique SA, CH
Ovitrelle	250 µg/0.5 mL	hCG	Recombinant	Merck Serono (Feltham, Middlesex, UK)

Table 1.
Analyzed products, batch numbers, and manufacturers' names of analyzed samples.

2.3 Chromatographic separation and detection

All separations were performed using the nanoRSLC UltiMate 3000 HPLC system coupled to the Q-Exactive Orbitrap Plus mass spectrometer (ThermoScientific, Vienna, Austria). Digested hCG and FSH were separated using trap column for sample loading and focusing (Acclaim PepMap C18, 300 µm ID × 5 mm, ThermoScientific, Vienna, Austria) and the pillar-arrayed-column (µPAC) with 2 µm interpillar distance and 2 m separation path (PharmaFluidics, Gent, Belgium) as the separation column. Both columns were operated in the column oven at 50°C. The sample was loaded onto the trap column using aqueous 0.01% HFBA at 30 µL/min and separated using the gradient generated by mixing mobile phases A (95% water, 5%AcN, and 0.1%FA) and B (50%AcN, 30%MeOH, 10% TFE, 10% water, and 0.1%FA).

Detection was performed using both UV at 214 nm and MS using positive electrospray ionization with a nanosource and ionization needle of 20 µm ID and 10 µm tip. The 20 most intensive signals in each MS scan were selected for MS/MS (fragmentation) with HCD at normalized collision energy (NCE) set to 30.

2.4 Data analysis

Raw data were transformed into Mascot generic files (MGF) for database search using MSConvert (www.proteowizzard.sourceforge.net). The database search was performed using the in-house Mascot server v.2.6 and the SwissProt database (status January 2018) using following parameters: trypsin was selected as enzyme, peptide mass precision was set to 10 ppm, carboxymethylation on Cys was selected as fixed modification and oxidation on Met, and phosphorylation on Ser, Thr, and Tyr were set as variable modifications.

Pathway analysis was performed using String (www.string-db.org).

3. Results

3.1 Identification of contaminant proteins in hCG preparations

All sample preparations were performed using standard procedures used in the Proteomics Core Facility of the Medical University of Vienna. No gel separations have been performed, and all results are generated upon the in-solution digest of different commercial formulations. Following chromatographic separation of tryptic peptides, the detection was performed using nanoelectrospray positive ionization and database search using the common SwissProt database.

For all analyzed samples, active substances were identified as major compounds. However, a number of other proteins were also identified in all samples. **Figure 1** shows an exemplary total ion chromatogram (TIC) of an hCG sample.

Table 2 shows the total number of identified compounds in each of the analyzed sample in addition to the main sample component, and an overview of the proteins with the highest scores identified in all samples is shown in **Table 3**.

3.2 Contaminant proteins in rhCG preparations versus uhCG

Recombinant hCG was significantly cleaner but a certain number of other proteins were also identified. Although the majority of these proteins seem to be

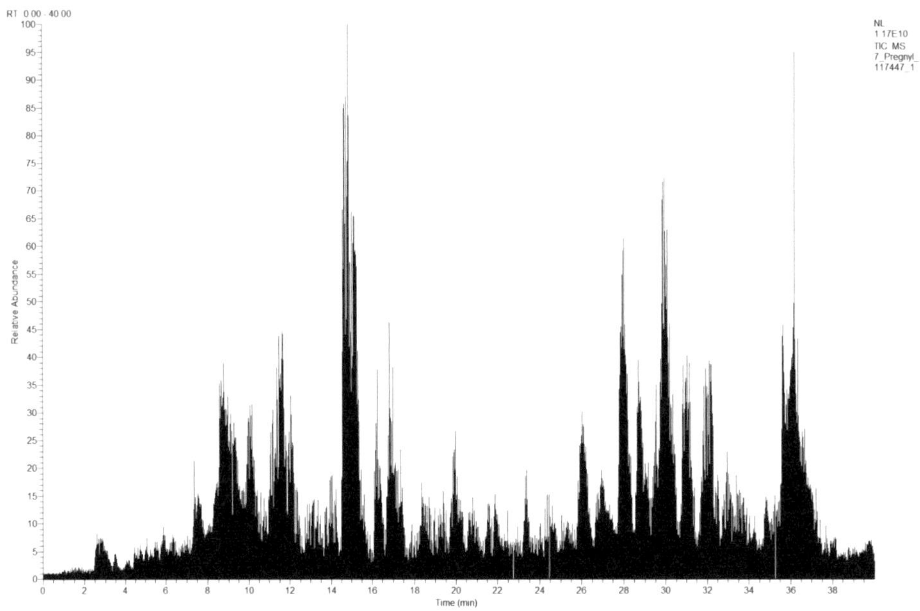

Figure 1.
Total ion chromatogram (TIC) of tryptic peptides generated from a Pregnyl formulation.

Sample's commercial name	Pregnyl	Chorimon	Ovitrelle
Number of analyzed batches	7	1	1
Origin	Urine	Urine	Recombinant
Number of additionally identified proteins	383	21	9

Table 2.
Total number of proteins identified in addition to the main therapeutic component in each of the samples' groups.

u-hCG	u-hCG-HP	r-hCG
Uromodulin	Growth/differentiation factor	Serum albumin
Ribonuclease pancreatic	Peptidoglycan recognition	Prelamin-A/C
Nonsecretory ribonuclease	Protein 1	Keratin, type I
Apolipoprotein D	Prostaglandin-H2 D-isomerase	cytoskeletal 9
Protein AMBP	Protein AMBP	Keratin, type I
Prothrombin	Bone marrow proteoglycan complement	cytoskeletal 10
Growth/differentiation factor 15	component C7	Keratin, type I
Insulin-like growth factor-binding	Neutrophil gelatinase-associated	cytoskeletal 14
protein 7	lipocalin	Histone H1.2
Cystatin-M	Serum albumin	Jupiter microtubule
Prostaglandin-H2 D-isomerase	Apolipoprotein D	associated
	Ribonuclease pancreatic	homolog 2
		Nucleoside
		diphosphate
		kinase A
		Keratin, type II
		cytoskeletal 1
		Trypsin-3

Table 3.
Proteins identified with highest scores in analyzed samples.

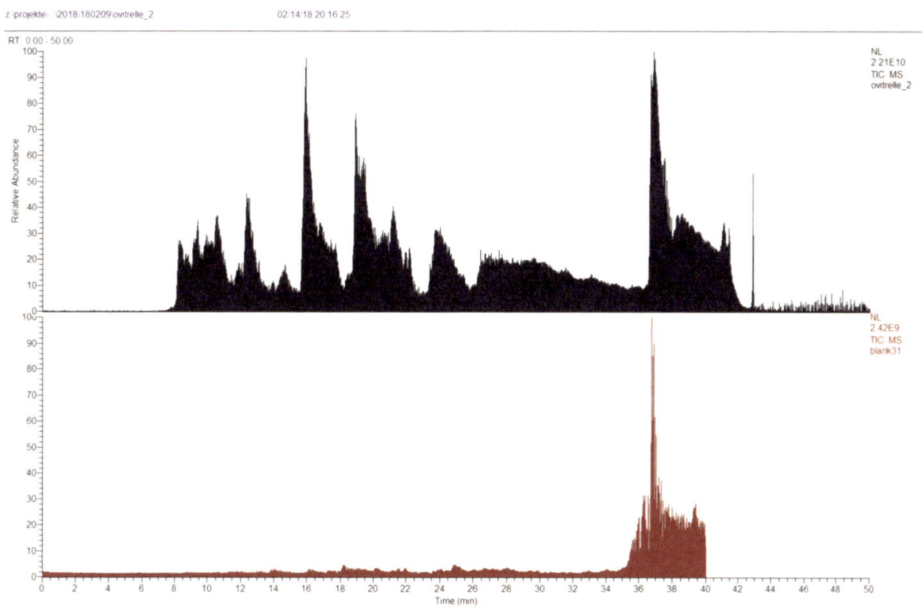

Figure 2.
Blank injection following analysis of digested recombinant hCG.

common contaminants such as keratins, in order to ensure that these proteins do not origin from previous injections of urinary formulations, blank sample injections (buffer used for dissolving peptides) were analyzed before and after the injection of each sample, and the TIC of such a blank injection is shown in **Figure 2**.

4. Discussion

In European Union, the production and the quality of medical products for both human and animal use is strongly regulated and controlled from both national health agencies and qualified bodies and from the European Medicines Agency. Companies producing medicines and medical devices must follow strict and detailed guidelines and secure that all operations are performed under governing GMP and GLP rules. These precautions shall secure the quality of the product and the safe use for the patients. Thennati et al. has described the method for the quality control of the recombinant product is ensured through analytical steps using SDS-gel separation and MALDI-ToF analysis of the final product [17]. Therefore, it was a great surprise to identify a number of proteins originating from the starting product (urine) in different batches of the final product.

A discussion on contaminant proteins in hCG formulations has already been published [4, 5, 7, 17–19], and several publications address the possibility of the presence of harmful substances in commercial formulation [13–15, 20–22] but no final decision was made and the urinary-derived hCG formulations are still widely used although it has been shown that recombinant hCG can be used with the same success rate.

Due to the lack of published data and reports on hCG formulations and the lack of information about these products, we have analyzed commercially available formulations that are routinely prescribed for patients undergoing IVF treatment.

The major active component, hCG, was identified in all analyzed samples and, in addition, human serum albumin (HSA), luteotropin subunit beta (LSHB), and glycoprotein hormones alpha chain (CGA). The presence of HSA in all samples can be explained by its secretion in urine and by the need of growing CHO cells, for recombinant hCG production, in culturing medium supplemented with HSA, which might contain a number of other proteins that were not removed when HSA purification was performed. The pathway and interaction analysis, shown in **Figure 3**, explains the dependence of co-expression between the hCG, LHB, and CGA and explains why these proteins can also be identified in recombinant products. Obviously, the production of hCG also induces the expression of other proteins involved in ovarian steroidogenesis, hormone activity, and regulation of hormone levels, which are identified with high confidence with MS/MS analysis. However, in this case, the identification of LHB is a false positive one, and we cannot claim that this protein is really present in the recombinant sample. The reason is that hCG and LHB have a common amino acid sequence between amino acids on positons 22

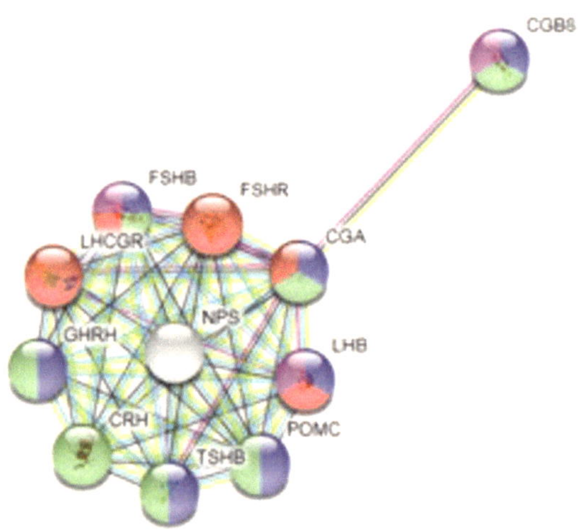

Figure 3.
Pathway describing the interdependence of hCG and LHB both of which were identified in recombinant products.

and 131 in the protein backbone. If other parts of the sequence cannot be identified, we cannot tell the proteins apart. However, in this case, the identification score and the identification of other amino acids in the hCG sequence show an unique identification.

4.1 Contaminant proteins in urinary-derived samples

As for the contaminants in urinary-derived products, uromodulin, which is also the major urinary protein, was a major hit following the major component. However, other proteins, such as alpha-1-microglobulin or apolipoprotein D, and prostaglandin were identified with high confidence. The contaminants in urinary-derived hCG formulations resemble urinary proteins identified in urine-only samples, which were described in a recently published study on stress-induced urinary incontinence [23].

Keratin was one of the major alien contaminants, and its presence suggests a contamination during the sample production and the origin might be the insufficient air-conditioning or the contamination of the packaging units, which might be traced back to the use of latex-made gloves, dust containing skin particles, etc. We can exclude the contamination in our lab since all sample preparation steps have been performed using the laminar flow and using nitrile gloves. The blank samples show no identifications of keratin or of other contaminations.

Additional distinction between the urinary and the recombinant products can be seen when looking at the GO analysis of the biological processes where these proteins are involved, as shown in **Figure 4**.

4.2 Contaminant proteins in recombinant samples

Products originating from the production process employing recombinant method have significantly less contaminant proteins of human origin. To our best knowledge, until now, there are no reports describing contaminations for recombinant hCG. Upon analysis, the hCG was the major component identified with contaminants such as keratin and human serum albumin (HSA). These contaminants are easy to explain, we have given an explanation for keratin in previous section, and HSA is most probably a contaminant from the culturing medium of CHO that was not completely removed upon hCG extraction.

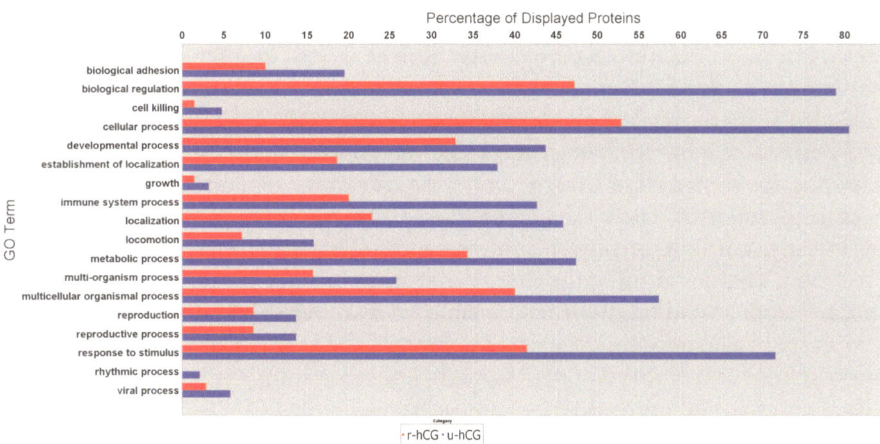

Figure 4.
GO term analysis of proteins identified in both urinary and recombinant formulations showing differences in their abundancies in biological processes.

4.3 Embryogenesis and hCG, influence of contaminants

Often, hCG is also known as “the hormone of pregnancy”. It plays an important part for establishing and maintaining pregnancy, and it is extensively used in IVF procedures. A serial measurement of hCG every 48 hours is being used to confirm the early pregnancy and to distinguish between normally progressing pregnancies from ectopic pregnancies or spontaneous abortions [10]. It was shown that the miscarriage rate is higher when assisted reproductive techniques (ARTs) are applied than with naturally occurring pregnancy [11]. Girard et al. evaluated the association between early β-hCG concentration increases, blastocyst morphology, and pregnancy evolution in a single-blastocyst transfer program. In most IVF laboratories, blastocyst transfers are associated with higher success rates of implantation as compared with the cleavage stage embryo as shown by Oron et al. [12] and Girard et al. [10]. Most laboratories report that blastocysts are selected for transfer according to their morphological characteristics. That means that physicians decide on implantation based on, that is, expansion degree, hatching status of the blastocysts, inner cell mass, or trophectoderm characteristics.

It is taught that hCG is involved in embryo implantation by modulating the activity of collagenases and plasminogen activators in an in-vitro system, as described by Yagel et al. [13]. Furthermore, it is an interesting and noteworthy feature that most of the mediators that have earlier been considered essential for the implantation process (i.e., EGF and IL-1/IL-6) are also involved in the regulation of hCG biosynthesis by the placental syncytiotrophoblasts [13–15] probably by modulating trophoblast differentiation. Therefore, Licht et al. postulated that hCG may play a central part in the hypothetical embryo-maternal cross talk and tested the hypothesis by simulating the effect of a very early pregnancy on the decidualized endometrium. The results suggested that, no immunoreactive hCG was found in the peripheral circulation (hCG<5 mIU/mL) and the treatment did not alter progesterone secretion by the corpus luteum, thus suggesting that the effects observed were direct.

As described in previous paragraph, urinary-derived hCG contains high number of contaminant proteins. Considering that, particularly, EGF is present in high concentrations in almost all tested commercial preparations of urinary-derived hCG, and additional experiments are needed to find out whether the effects observed are due to hCG or to a contamination from the formulation.

Furthermore, contaminant proteins identified in hCG formulations can be the source of severe allergic reactions and can also trigger immune response that must not necessarily been manifested externally; however, it can negatively affect embryo implantation and embryogenesis. Koh et al. [16] and Phipps et.al [17] described the cases of IgE-mediated immunoreaction after intramuscular administration of urinary-derived gonadotropins. This type of allergic reactions occurs shortly after administration of urinary-derived gonadotropin, and it occurs with symptoms like shortness of breath, wheezing, flushing, general weakness, and dizziness. In all reported cases, the IgE-mediated allergic reaction could be confirmed after intradermal skin testing with the same uhCG lot. Testing with rhCG triggered no reaction, thus confirming the theory that some urinary proteins can trigger an immune response and might be responsible for anaphylactic reactions. Immune reaction could also influence the development of the embryo and hinder normal embryogenesis and embryo implantation in endometrium.

Kajihara et al. [18] proposed that some urinary-derived hCG (uhCG) impurities like EDN or ribonuclease 2 could influence inflammatory and immunological processes through regulation of apoptosis in endometrial cells and, therefore, directly influence embryo nesting and development during IVF. Considering that some patients undergo lengthy and intensive treatment with uhCG, an effect cannot be excluded.

Uromodulin, as the most abundant protein in human urine, is also detected in various uhCG formulations as the most abundant one. Uromodulin has been described as a powerful stimulator of the immune system through its ability to bind on the surface of almost all blood cells and to encourage the cellular production of cytokines, increase lymphocyte proliferation and phagocytosis [19, 20]. Using a mouse model, de Silva Antunes et al. suggested that uromodulin, but also some other urinary proteins, that is, major urinary proteins [13, 14, 17] or kidney androgen-regulated protein act as a possible allergens in the T-cell-mediated allergic reaction [21]. Otherwise, Phinuster et al. [22] suggested protective role of uromodulin in amniotic fluid in the fetus defense against anti-allogenic antibodies and immunosuppressive effect on T-cell-mediated allogenic rejection.

5. Conclusion

Formulations of hCG, both urinary and recombinant, contain contaminant proteins that originate from either starting material or has been introduced during the manufacturing process. The information about these contaminants cannot be identified on products' leaflets.

We could show that urinary-derived products contain a significant number of human proteins that obviously originate from the starting raw material—the human urine.

We think that this issue must be approached and discussed since the recombinant proteins show no such contamination and their use has been proven safe and effective.

Due to an important role played by hCG in embryo development in healthy subjects and embryo implantation during the IVF procedure, it is of great importance to thoroughly check the quality of the formulations and apply production steps for the best possible removal of all contaminant proteins from the final product and prevent possible adverse and allergic reactions, which might affect embryogenesis in general and embryo implantation in uterus.

Author details

Tanja Panić-Janković[1] and Goran Mitulović[1,2]*

1 Clinical Department of Laboratory Medicine, Medical University of Vienna, Vienna, Austria

2 Proteomic Core Facility, Medical University of Vienna, Vienna, Austria

*Address all correspondence to: goran.mitulovic@meduniwien.ac.at

References

[1] Chang P, Kenley S, Burns T, Denton G, Currie K, DeVane G, et al. Recombinant human chorionic gonadotropin (rhCG) in assisted reproductive technology: Results of a clinical trial comparing two doses of rhCG (OvidrelR) to urinary hCG (ProfasiR) for induction of final follicular maturation in in vitro fertilization–embryo transfer. Fertility and Sterility. 2001;**76**(1):67-74

[2] Tsampalas M, Gridelet V, Berndt S, Foidart J-M, Geenen V, d'Hauterive SP. Human chorionic gonadotropin: A hormone with immunological and angiogenic properties. Journal of Reproductive Immunology. 2010;**85**(1):93-98

[3] Licht P, Losch A, Dittrich R, Neuwinger J, Siebzehnrubl E, Wildt L. Novel insights into human endometrial paracrinology and embryo-maternal communication by intrauterine microdialysis. Human Reproduction Update. 1998;**4**(5):532-538

[4] Balasch J, Peñarrubia J, Fábregues F, Vidal E, Casamitjana R, Manau D, et al. Ovarian responses to recombinant FSH or HMG in normogonadotropic women following pituitary desensitisation by a depot GnRH agonist for assisted reproduction. Reproductive Biomedicine Online. 2003;7:35-42

[5] Ludwig M, Doody KJ, Doody KM. Use of recombinant human chorionic gonadotropin in ovulation induction. Fertility and Sterility. 2003;**79**(5):1051-1059

[6] Hugues JN. Comparative use of urinary and recombinant human chorionic gonadotropins in women. Treatments in Endocrinology. 2004;**3**(6):371-379

[7] Al-Inany H, Aboulghar MA, Mansour RT, Proctor M. Recombinant versus urinary gonadotrophins for triggering ovulation in assisted conception. Human Reproduction. 2005;**20**(8):2061-2073

[8] Buhler K, Fischer R. Recombinant human LH supplementation versus supplementation with urinary hCG-based LH activity during controlled ovarian stimulation in the long GnRH-agonist protocol: A matched case–control study. Gynecological Endocrinology. 2012;**28**:345-350

[9] Eftekhar M, Khalili MA, Rahmani E. The efficacy of recombinant versus urinary HCG in ART outcome. Iranian Journal of Reproductive Medicine. 2012;**10**(6):543-548

[10] Girard J-M, Simorre M, Leperlier F, Reignier A, Lefebvre T, Barrière P, et al. Association between early βhCG kinetics, blastocyst morphology and pregnancy outcome in a single-blastocyst transfer program. European Journal of Obstetrics & Gynecology and Reproductive Biology. 2018;**225**:189-193

[11] Ochsenkühn R, Arzberger A, Von Schönfeldt V, Engel J, Thaler CJ, Noss U. Predictive value of early serum β-hCG levels after single blastocyst transfer. Acta Obstetricia et Gynecologica Scandinavica. 2009;**88**(12):1382-1388

[12] Oron G, Esh-Broder E, Son W-Y, Holzer H, Tulandi T. Predictive value of maternal serum human chorionic gonadotropin levels in pregnancies achieved by in vitro fertilization with single cleavage and single blastocyst embryo transfers. Fertility and Sterility. 2015;**103**(6):1526-1531. e2

[13] Yagel S, Geva TE, Solomon H, Shimonovitz S, Reich R, Finci-Yeheskel

Z, et al. High levels of human chorionic gonadotropin retard first trimester trophoblast invasion in vitro by decreasing urokinase plasminogen activator and collagenase activities. The Journal of Clinical Endocrinology & Metabolism. 1993;**77**(6):1506-1511

[14] Harty JR, Kauma SW. Interleukin-1 beta stimulates colony-stimulating factor-1 production in placental villous core mesenchymal cells. The Journal of Clinical Endocrinology & Metabolism. 1992;**75**(3):947-950

[15] Sawai K, Matsuzaki N, Kameda T, Hashimoto K, Okada T, Shimoya K, et al. Leukemia inhibitory factor produced at the fetomaternal interface stimulates chorionic gonadotropin production: Its possible implication during pregnancy, including implantation period. The Journal of Clinical Endocrinology & Metabolism. 1995;**80**(4):1449-1456

[16] Koh YI, Choi IS, Lee H-C, Na H-S, Oh S-T. Desensitization to urine-derived gonadotropins in a woman with secondary infertility. Annals of Allergy, Asthma & Immunology. 2001;**87**(5):434-438

[17] Phipps WR, Holden D, Sheehan RK. Use of recombinant human follicle-stimulating hormone for in vitro fertilization-embryo transfer after severe systemic immunoglobulin E-mediated reaction to urofollitropin. Fertility and Sterility. 1996;**66**(1):148-150

[18] Kajihara T, Tochigi H, Uchino S, Itakura A, Brosens JJ, Ishihara O. Differential effects of urinary and recombinant chorionic gonadotropin on oxidative stress responses in decidualizing human endometrial stromal cells. Placenta. 2011;**32**(8):592-597

[19] Su S-J, Yeh T-M. The dynamic responses of pro-inflammatory and anti-inflammatory cytokines of human mononuclear cells induced by uromodulin. Life Sciences. 1999;**65**(24):2581-2590

[20] Yu C-L, Lin W-M, Liao T-S, Tsai C-Y, Sun K-H, Chen K-H. Tamm-Horsfall glycoprotein (THG) purified from normal human pregnancy urine increases phagocytosis, complement receptor expressions and arachidonic acid metabolism of polymorphonuclear neutrophils. Immunopharmacology. 1992;**24**(3):181-190

[21] da Silva Antunes R, Pham J, McMurtrey C, Hildebrand WH, Phillips E, Mallal S, et al. Urinary peptides as a novel source of T cell allergen epitopes. Frontiers in Immunology. 2018;**9**:886

[22] Phinuster GM, Marshall RD. Tamm-Horsfall glycoprotein in human amniotic fluid. Clinica Chimica Acta. 1983;**128**(2):261-269

[23] Koch M, Mitulovic G, Hanzal E, Umek W, Seyfert S, Mohr T, et al. Urinary proteomic pattern in female stress urinary incontinence: A pilot study. International Urogynecology Journal. 2016;**27**(11):1729-1734

Chapter 3

Clinical Application of In Vitro Maturation of Oocytes

Xiaolin La, Jing Zhao and Zhihui Wang

Abstract

In vitro maturation (IVM) is a technique used to induce immature oocytes collected in different periods of embryonic growth. The rates vary for immature oocytes collected from different clinical sources to potentially develop into embryos and achieve live birth. As an effective treatment method, IVM can be used to treat patients with polycystic ovary syndrome (PCOS), ovarian hyperresponsiveness, and hyporesponsiveness, as well as to preserve the fertility of cancer patients. This technology has been used worldwide for the birth of thousands of healthy babies. The improvement in clinical IVM technology mainly focuses on the IVM medium and the optimization of the culture environment and operation process. At present, with the improvement in the in vitro fertilization (IVF) efficiency and culture systems, a natural cycle or mild stimulation may be more suitable for women receiving IVF treatments. A new treatment option was proposed to combine natural cycle/ mild stimulation IVF with IVM. In particular, the combination of mild stimulation IVF and IVM is not only expected to become a viable alternative to current standard treatments but may also become a potential option of first-line treatment.

Keywords: in vitro maturation (IVM), assisted reproductive technologies (ARTs), cytoplasmic maturation, antral follicles, granulosa cells

1. Introduction

In the 1960s, major milestones were achieved in in vitro maturation (IVM) of human oocytes, and in vitro fertilization (IVF) of IVM oocytes was also established. Therefore, modern assisted reproductive technologies (ARTs) are based on IVM. Currently, the clinical application of IVM may be extended to treat patients with polycystic ovary syndrome (PCOS), ovarian hyperresponsiveness, and hyporesponsiveness, as well as to preserve the fertility of cancer patients [1]. In 2013, the practice committees of the American Society for Reproductive Medicine (ASRM) and the Society for Assisted Reproductive Technology (SART) stated that the clinical pregnancy rate of IVM was still lower than that of conventional IVF, and hence IVM could not yet be considered the first treatment choice for all cases of female infertility [2].

The current standard protocol for ovulation induction in clinical practice involves intense stimulation with nonphysiological doses of gonadotropins to obtain an average of 10–15 or even dozens of mature oocytes per woman. Although the regimen of high-dose gonadotropin treatment may enable the retrieval of a larger number of oocytes, this approach can exert several short- and long-term adverse effects, including the risk of ovarian hyperstimulation syndrome (OHSS).

IntechOpen

At present, with the improvement in the IVF efficiency and culture systems, a natural cycle or mild stimulation may be more suitable for women receiving IVF treatments. A previous study showed that natural cycle or mild stimulation IVF is more effective than conventional stimulation protocols in patients with a low functional ovarian reserve [3]. In contrast to the standard stimulation protocol, the mild stimulation protocol is a safer and more rational regimen that helps reduce the hormone dosage, lower treatment risks, and retrieve a small number of high-quality oocytes. Despite these theoretical advantages, the mild stimulation protocol has yet to become a mainstream treatment modality in the United States. With the development of IVM technology, a modified protocol able to increase the success rates of natural cycle or mild stimulation IVF has been established. In this protocol, in addition to the retrieval of mature oocytes in naturally or mildly stimulated cycles, immature oocytes from small follicles are also retrieved for IVM, thereby increasing the total number of retrieved oocytes in a single treatment cycle and the clinical pregnancy rate. Data from previous clinical studies has shown that the combined use of natural cycle or mild stimulation IVF with IVM can expand the applicable scope of IVM technology to the treatment of various types of female infertility and has resulted in satisfactory clinical pregnancy rates and live birth rates [4, 5].

2. Mechanism of oocyte maturation

Cyclic adenosine monophosphate (cAMP) plays an important role in regulating the maturation of oocytes. The mural granulosa cells (MGC) located on the follicular wall contain natriuretic peptide precursor C (NPPC), while the cumulus cells around oocytes express natriuretic peptide receptor 2 (NPR2). Oocyte-derived paracrine factors can promote the activation of NPR2 in cumulus cells, while the NPPC in mural granulosa cells can bind to NPR2 receptors in cumulus cells to produce cyclic guanosine monophosphate (cGMP), which then enters into oocytes through gap junctions to inhibit the activity of phosphodiesterase (PDE3A), thereby maintaining a high level of cAMP in oocytes and the arrest of oocytes in the meiosis cycle. The activation of PDE3A by luteinizing hormone (LH) downregulates the level of cAMP in oocytes and induces the maturation of oocytes, thereby relieving the immature oocytes in the germinal vesicle (GV) stage or first meiotic metaphase (MII) from cell cycle arrest, so that they can complete the first meiosis and enter the second MII to develop into mature oocytes [6]. Zhang et al. [7] reported that estradiol can promote and maintain the expression of NPR2 in cumulus cells and participate in NPPC-mediated meiotic arrest of oocytes in vitro. These studies have opened up a new field of molecular mechanistic research on resuming the meiosis of oocytes, providing a theoretical basis for revealing the molecular mechanisms underlying the maturation of oocytes.

Studies have found that small molecule ribonucleotides (microRNAs) are also important for oocyte maturation. A certain number of dynamic and stable microRNAs were found in both mature oocytes and early-stage embryos, presumably contributing to the maturation of oocytes. Kim et al. [8, 9] reported that microRNAs may affect oocyte maturation by altering the gene expression and function of cumulus cells through cumulus cell interaction and paracrine secretion. Let-7 is one of the most abundant microRNAs in the ovary. Upregulation of Let-7c can increase the rate of oocyte maturation, suggesting that Let-7c may be involved in the information exchange between oocytes and surrounding mural granulosa cells. In addition, maturation-promoting factor (MPF), cytostatic factor (CSF), oocyte maturation inhibitor (OMI), and mitogen-activated protein kinase (MAPK) are involved in oocyte maturation and division [7]. The mechanisms underlying oocyte maturation awaits further studies.

3. Definition of oocyte IVM

The biological definition of oocyte IVM is to remove immature oocytes in the GV stage from antral follicles and culture them in a suitable culture system, so that these immature oocytes can mature to MII stage in vitro. However, the clinical definition of IVM technology for immature human oocytes is completely different from its biological definition. The differences include the different sources of immature oocytes, the different protocols used to induce ovulation, and the different time of oocyte retrieval. These factors may lead to the situation where the immature oocytes retrieved clinically are not in the GV stage. The use of human chorionic gonadotropin (hCG) to induce ovulation prior to clinical retrieval of oocytes may lead to the initiation of endogenous oocyte maturation, and hence some of the retrieved immature oocytes may have undergone germinal vesicle breakdown (GVBD) or entered the MI stage. Although immature oocytes in the MI stage have initiated the process of in vivo maturation, they still need to participate in the procedure of in vitro culture and maturation. Therefore, the definition of clinical IVM treatment should include the in vitro culture of immature oocytes in the GV and MI stages.

A recent point of view proposed to give the clinical definition of IVM of immature oocytes based on the diameter of follicles when the oocytes are retrieved [10]. However, this definition is not completely scientific, since the meiotic state of oocytes cannot be completely determined according to the size of follicles during the stimulation cycle [11, 12]. In addition, for immature oocytes collected from different clinical sources, their maturation rate and the rates to potentially develop into embryos and achieve live birth are different. Therefore, for clinical definition and research of IVM, attention should be paid to the effect of different sources of immature oocytes on the efficiency of IVM.

4. Factors affecting the in vitro maturation of oocytes

4.1 Effect of culture time on in vitro maturation of oocytes

Maturation of oocytes includes the nuclear and cytoplasmic maturation of oocytes. Nuclear maturation refers to the rupture of the germinal vesicle, separation of homologous chromosomes, appearance of the perivitelline space, and discharge of the first polar body. Cytoplasmic maturation refers to the completion of protein phosphorylation and dephosphorylation as well as the rearrangement of organelles in oocytes. Only the oocytes whose nucleus and cytoplasm are matured simultaneously can have adequate fertility and the potential for embryo development. Studies have found that most oocytes cultured in vitro can reach maturity within 24–48 h. The length of in vitro culture can affect the developmental potential of the embryo. The rate of nuclear maturation in oocytes cultured for 48 h in vitro is significantly higher than that for 24 h, but the rate of cytoplasmic maturation in oocytes cultured for 48 h is not significantly different from that for 24 h. Excessive culture time leads to the aging of oocytes and an increased level of associated genetic risks. When the culture time is too short, the maturation of cytoplasm and nucleus is not synchronized and will affect the subsequent development potential of the embryo. Wrenzycki et al. [13] found that oocytes only possess the ability to mature in the final stage of development. Therefore, adequate extension of IVM time can promote the necessary process of oocyte maturation, increase the rate of nuclear maturation in immature oocytes, and significantly improve in vitro developmental potential of oocytes and the rate of high-quality embryos.

4.2 Effects of hormones on in vitro maturation of oocytes

Gonadotropin can promote the expansion of cumulus cells and stimulate the maturation of the nucleus and cytoplasm of oocytes, thus facilitating the formation of embryos and blastocysts in the cleavage stage and playing an important role in follicular development [14]. The addition of follicle-stimulating hormone to the culture medium for oocyte maturation can promote the cytoplasmic maturation of oocytes. Some scholars believe that the effect of follicle-stimulating hormone is related to its concentration. When the concentration is 5 g/mL, a relatively high cleavage rate (79.1%) and blastocyst rate (16.1%) can be obtained [15]. The addition of LH or human chorionic gonadotropin to the IVM culture medium may promote protein synthesis, enhance oocyte metabolism, and facilitate oocyte maturation. The concentration of estradiol (E2) in the human body increases with an increasing volume of follicles. In addition, estradiol is involved in maintaining the meiotic arrest of oocytes and can promote the cytoplasmic maturation of oocytes. During in vitro culture of oocytes, nuclear maturation is faster than cytoplasmic maturation. Therefore, the addition of E2 to the culture medium helps synchronize the development of the nucleus and cytoplasm in oocytes.

4.3 Effect of antioxidant addition on in vitro maturation of oocytes

As a hydrophobic activator, forskolin (FSK) can increase the activity of adenylate cyclase in mammalian cells and the level of intracellular cAMP. By adding FSK to an IVM culture medium, Ezoe et al. [16] significantly improved the developmental capacity of oocytes in the GV stage. By adding FSK to the culture medium, Zeng et al. [17] promoted the synchronization of nuclear and cytoplasmic maturation and increased the rates of maturation, cleavage, and high-quality embryos. During IVM, the presence of oxidative stress may block oocyte maturation, lead to abnormal gene expression, and impair the cytoplasmic and nuclear development of oocytes, thereby resulting in the failure to obtain high-quality oocytes and decreasing the fertility and developmental capacity. The addition of antioxidants to the culture medium can reduce the damage caused by oxidative stress. By adding a-lipoic acid to the culture medium, Zavareh et al. [18] reduced the content of active oxygen, increased the total antioxidation capacity, and promoted the nuclear and cytoplasmic maturation of oocytes in vitro. The results of Mokhber et al. [19, 20] showed that an appropriate concentration of a natural antioxidant, crocin (100 g/mL), and aqueous extract of saffron (40 g/mL) can increase the concentration of glutathione (GSH), protect oocytes, and significantly increase IVM rate and fertility rate.

4.4 Effect of co-culture with mural granulosa cells on in vitro maturation of oocytes

Together with cumulus cells and follicular fluid, MGC form an in vivo environment for oocyte maturation. Co-culture with MGC can increase the rate of nuclear and cytoplasmic maturation of immature oocytes. Studies have shown that co-culture with parietal MGC can improve the nuclear maturation of naked oocytes, slow down the nuclear maturation of naked oocytes, increase the content of glutathione in naked oocytes, reduce the activity of glucose-6-phosphate dehydrogenase in naked oocytes, increase the rate of cytoplasmic maturation, and facilitate the simultaneous development of the nucleus and cytoplasm of oocytes [21]. Although immature oocytes detached of MGC can still mature, they cannot undergo normal fertilization and development because the cytoplasm is not synchronously matured [22]. The addition of a certain amount of MGC to the culture medium can delay the nuclear maturation of oocytes, so that the maturation of the nucleus and cytoplasm becomes more synchronized. However, there is currently no uniform standard for the amount of MGC addition. Choi et al. [23] significantly increased the development potential of embryos by co-culturing the oocyte-corona-cumulus complex with naked oocytes at a 1:5 ratio.

4.5 Effect of co-culture with oviductal epithelial cells on in vitro maturation of oocytes

Some scholars have pointed out that the maturation of oocytes is completed in the fallopian tube, and hence some components of the fallopian tube may affect the maturation process of oocytes. Human tubal fluid (HTF) has been used to culture oocytes. Shirazi et al. [24] co-cultured ovine oocytes with oviductal epithelial cells (OECs) and conducted IVF, resulting in higher cleavage and blastocyst rates.

4.6 Effect of co-culture with mesenchymal stem cells on in vitro maturation of oocytes

In addition to the potential of self-renewal and multidirectional differentiation, mesenchymal stem cells (MSCs) can also secrete a variety of cytokines and growth factors, and some biologically active factors can enhance the in vitro maturation of oocytes and subsequent developmental potential of embryos. By adding MSCs to a culture medium, Ling et al. [25] significantly increased the maturation rate and rate of blastocyst formation of immature murine oocytes. It can be seen that the co-culture system with MSCs can promote the simultaneous development of the nucleus and cytoplasm of murine oocytes.

5. Sources of immature oocytes

5.1 Oocyte retrieval from cesarean section or gynecological surgery

Immature oocytes retrieved from the ovarian cortex during cesarean section can be cultured in vitro to achieve maturation, fertilization, and healthy progeny. The mature oocytes cultured in this way are expected to be used as the source of oocytes to preserve female fertility [26]. At present, few studies have investigated the approach to obtain immature oocytes during cesarean section for in vitro culture, and hence more studies are needed to prove the safety and effectiveness of immature oocytes obtained from cesarean section.

In addition to cesarean section, immature oocytes can also be obtained via gynecological surgery in the follicular phase or luteal phase. The number of retrieved oocytes is mainly related to the age, pathological status, and stage of the menstrual cycle of the patient. Clinical studies have confirmed that oocyte retrieval carried out at different stages of the menstrual cycle does not affect the rate of in vitro maturation and the rate of fertilization of oocytes, suggesting that IVM technique can be used to preserve fertility in cancer patients during the follicular phase or luteal phase [27]. Therefore, for cancer patients who lack sufficient time for treatment and are unable to use hormone to induce ovulation, immature oocytes can be retrieved before chemotherapy to carry out IVM and vitrification to maximize the preservation of fertility.

5.2 PCOS patients

A large number of antral follicles are present in the ovary of infertile women with anovulatory PCOS. These antral follicles are more sensitive to gonadotropins, and hence the risk of OHSS is increased when hormones are used to induce ovulation. Therefore, for PCOS patients, immature oocytes can be retrieved from antral follicle for in vitro maturation [28]. The use of hCG at 36 h before oocyte retrieval in PCOS patients can promote the resumption of meiosis of immature oocytes and their in vitro maturation, improving the rate of pregnancy and clinical outcomes [29]. The use of small doses of gonadotropin before the retrieval of immature oocytes from PCOS patients is also beneficial to improve the maturation potential of oocytes, increasing the rate of embryo implantation and clinical pregnancy. In addition, IVM techniques can also be considered for some PCOS patients with no or low response to hormones [30].

5.3 Women with normal ovaries and menstrual cycles

Based on the advantages of low hormone dosage, low cost, and simple treatment process, IVM has been gradually applied to the treatment of infertile women with normal ovaries and regular menstrual cycles. However, it remains controversial as whether the use of hCG is required in the IVM treatment of this type of patient prior to oocyte retrieval. It should be noted that the hCG trigger exerts different effects on normal ovaries and PCOS patients. In the IVM treatment cycle of PCOS patients, dominant follicles are barely visible in the ovary, but MI-stage oocytes can be retrieved from small follicles after hCG-induced ovulation. However, after the hCG trigger is used in the normal ovary during the follicular phase, most oocytes retrieved from small follicles are oocytes in the GV stage. There is currently no evidence suggesting that the hCG trigger exerts a significant effect on the pregnancy rate, live birth rate, or abortion rate in the IVM of immature oocytes obtained from normal ovaries [31]. However, the accuracy of these findings is limited by the small number of samples. Therefore, a well-designed, randomized, and controlled clinical trial is needed to further confirm the optimal dosage and timing of hCG administration.

6. IVM culture system

6.1 Improvement of IVM media

The in vitro maturation of oocytes is mainly affected by culture conditions. At present, the common media used for the IVM of immature human oocytes include TCM-199 medium, Ham's F10 medium, and Chang's medium. In addition, serum, gonadotropin [follicle-stimulating hormone and luteinizing hormone], growth factors, and steroids can be added in a basal medium to produce a complex medium. At present, commercial IVM media have been widely used. However, no breakthrough has been made in the research on improving the quality of oocytes by improving the IVM medium. In recent years, research and application of antioxidants and growth-promoting factors have promoted the advancement of this technology to some extent. In addition, using cell cycle regulators or inhibitors of mitotic spindle formation, the synchronization of nuclear and cytoplasmic maturation of immature oocytes can be achieved by inhibiting GVBD, thereby increasing the blastocyst rate and live birth rate in animal models [32]. However, the safety and efficacy of this method in human oocytes should be further verified.

6.2 Optimization of IVM culture environment and process

The culture environment, equipment, and related operations in the IVM system may affect the in vitro maturation and embryo development of immature oocytes. Therefore, the optimization of the embryo culture environment and process of in vitro operation will help to maintain the potential of embryonic development [33, 34]. The three-dimensional culture system can support the development of follicles by using biological materials to maintain cell-to-cell information exchange. In addition, mature oocytes can be obtained by using a three-dimensional culture system in the in vitro culture of anterior follicles of nonhuman primates [35], although no reports are available regarding the use of a three-dimensional culture system in the in vitro culture of immature human oocytes. A past study has used microreactors to form three-dimensional bioreactors to support the growth of different types of cells [36]. Consisting of a drop of liquid encapsulated by hydrophobic powder particles, this system can provide a suitable microenvironment for in vitro maturation of oocytes. In addition, the development of microfluidic technology will exert an important impact in the field of human gametes and preimplantation embryo development and will have potential applications in the field of ART. This technology enables the creation of microfluidic models mimicking the "menstrual cycle of women" [37]. These models include interconnected 3D models of different tissues, such as 3D models of the ovaries, fallopian tubes, uterus, cervix, and vagina, in the female reproductive system and the endocrine cycle between various organ modules. The mechanical and biochemical properties of microfluidic systems still require intensive research before these systems can be applied to clinical applications in areas such as IVM of immature human oocytes.

7. Clinical application and safety of IVM

At present, the in vitro maturation rate of immature human oocytes can reach 70%, but the developmental potential of mature oocytes obtained in vitro is still lower than that of mature oocytes obtained in vivo. In addition, the rate of blastocyst development and the rate of implantation are relatively low after the fertilization of IVM oocytes. The main reason of such discrepancy may be related to non-synchronized nuclear and cytoplasmic maturation during IVM. With the further development in the basic and clinical research of IVM, the in-depth study on the mechanisms of oocyte maturation and mastery of key factors involved in oocyte maturation will contribute to the improvement and optimization of clinical IVM technology.

The results of current research showed that human oocytes matured in vivo or in vitro display no significant differences in terms of their spindle morphology, organelle distribution, cortical particle distribution, and mitochondrial morphology [38, 39]. By observing embryos dynamically using time-lapse videos, it was confirmed that oocytes matured in vivo or in vitro showed no significant differences in terms of the morphological dynamics observed during the early development of embryos derived from these oocytes [40]. Another study has also shown that the oocytes matured in vitro and in vivo are different in terms of their organelle function, distribution, and gene expression [41]. The different experimental conclusions mentioned above may be caused by different sources and quality of oocytes used in these studies. Therefore, attention should be paid to clarify the IVM efficiency of oocytes retrieved from different sources, so as to reasonably evaluate the safety of IVM. In terms of epigenetics, a study has reported that IVM exerts no significant effect on the methylation level of maternal imprinted genes, such as

LIT1, SNRPN, PEG3, and GTL2, in human oocytes [42]. After an imprinted gene examination was carried out for infant chorionic cells and cord blood obtained from IVM and a standard stimulation protocol, no significant difference was observed between the two methods [43, 44]. Currently, the follow-up of IVM-aided pregnancies shows that the IVM technique does not increase the risk of pregnancy, the rate of maternal complications, and the rate of neonatal abnormalities [45, 46]. However, due to a small sample size and the lack of in-depth study on epigenetics, the clinical application and safety of IVM still require investigations of large sample sizes to reach a definitive conclusion regarding the safety of IVM in terms of epigenetics.

At present, more than 5000 IVM babies have been born worldwide, and the rate of clinical pregnancy among PCOS patients undergoing IVM treatment can reach about 35–40% [47]. IVM has been extended from the basic research to the treatment of patients with PCOS, ovarian hyperresponsiveness and hyporesponsiveness, as well as cancer patients to preserve the fertility. Therefore, IVM has a prospect of broad applications.

8. Conclusion

At present, the application scope of IVM technology can be extended to patients with various causes of infertility. In addition, the IVM technology is associated with acceptable pregnancy and live birth rates. Although IVM has been used as an effective treatment and achieved significant outcomes with thousands of healthy IVM babies having been delivered, IVM is still considered as an experimental technique by the society. With the development of IVM technology, the combination of natural cycle IVF with the IVM of immature oocytes can be used as an attractive regimen to promote IVM treatment. More infertile women can benefit from such approaches if the treatment process is simplified by mild stimulation, especially when the difficulty to obtain immature oocytes is reduced. Therefore, the combination of mild stimulation IVF and IVM treatment can become a viable alternative to current standard treatments. With the accumulation of more experience and results, it will be further demonstrated that the combination of mild stimulation IVF and IVM is not only a viable alternative to current standard treatments but may also become a potential option of first-line treatment.

Author details

Xiaolin La*, Jing Zhao and Zhihui Wang
First Affiliated Hospital of Xinjiang Medical University, Xinjiang, China

*Address all correspondence to: 909232905@qq.com

References

[1] Sauerbrun-Cutler MT, Vega M, Keltz M. et al., In vitro maturation and its role in clinical assisted reproductive technology. Obstetrical & Gynecological Survey. 2015;**70**(1):45-57

[2] Practice Committees of the American Society for Reproductive Medicine and the Society for Assisted Reproductive Technology. In vitro maturation: A committee opinion. Fertility and Sterility. 2013;**99**(3):663-666

[3] Xu Y, Li J, Zhou G, et al. Clinical outcomes for various causes of infertility with natural-cycle in vitro fertilization combined with in vitro maturation of immature oocytes. Fertility and Sterility. 2010;**94**(2):777-780

[4] Chian RC, Cao YX. In vitro maturation of immature human oocytes for clinical application. Methods in Molecular Biology. 2014;**1154**:271-288

[5] Yang SH, Patrizio P, Yoon SH, et al. Comparison of pregnancy outcomes in natural cycle IVF/M treatment with or without mature oocytes retrieved at time of egg collection. Systems Biology in Reproductive Medicine. 2012;**58**(3):154-159

[6] Zhang M, Su Y, Sugiura K, et al. Granulosa cell ligand NPPC and its receptor NPR 2 maintain meiotic arrest in mouse oocytes. Science. 2010;**330**(62):366-369

[7] Zhang M, Su Y, Sugiura K, et al. Estradiol promotes and maintains cumulus cell expression of natriuretic peptide receptor 2 (NPR 2) and meiotic arrest in mouse oocytes in vitro. Endocrinology. 2011;**152**(11):4377-4385

[8] Gilchrist GC, Tscherner A, Nalpathamkalam T, et al. MicroRNA expression during bovine oocyte maturation and fertilization. International Journal of Molecular Sciences. 2016;**17**(3):396

[9] Kim YJ, Ku SY, Kim YY, et al. MicroRNAs transfected into granulosa cells may regulate oocyte meiotic competence during in vitro maturation of mouse follicles. Human Reproduction. 2013;**28**(11):3050-3061

[10] Dahan MH, Tan SL, Chung J, et al. Clinical definition paper on in vitro maturation of human oocytes. Human Reproduction. 2016;**31**(7):1383-1386

[11] Coticchio G. IVM in need of clear definitions. Human Reproduction. 2016;**31**(7):1387-1389

[12] De Vos M, Smitz J, Thompson JG, et al. The definition of IVM is clear-variations need defining. Human Reproduction. 2016;**31**(11):2411-2415

[13] Wrenzycki C, Stinshoff H. Maturation environment and impact on subsequent developmental competence of bovine oocytes. Reproduction in Domestic Animals. 2013;**48**(Suppl 1): 38-43

[14] Grynberg M, Poulain M, Le Parco S, et al. Similar in vitro maturation rates of oocytes retrieved during the follicular or luteal phase offer flexible options for urgent fertility preservation in breast cancer patients. Human Reproduction. 2016;**31**(3):623-629

[15] Pereira GR, Lorenzo PL, Carneiro GF, et al. Influence of equine growth hormone, insulin-like growth factor-1 and its interaction with gonadotropins on in vitro maturation and cytoskeleton morphology in equine oocytes. Animal. 2013;7(9):1493-1499

[16] Ezoe K, Yabuuchi A, Tani T, et al. Developmental competence of vitrified-warmed bovine oocytes at the germinal-vesicle stage is improved by cyclic

adenosine monophosphate modulators during in vitro maturation. PLoS One. 2015;**10**(5):e0126801

[17] Zeng H, Ren Z, Guzman L, et al. Heparin and cAMP modulators interact during pre-in vitro maturation to affect mouse and human oocyte meiosis and developmental competence. Human Reproduction. 2013;**28**(6):1536-1545

[18] Zavareh S, Karimi I, Salehnia M, et al. Effect of in vitro maturation technique and alpha lipoic acid supplementation on oocyte maturation rate: Focus on oxidative status of oocytes. International Journal of Fertility and Sterility. 2016;**9**(4):442-451

[19] Mokhber Maleki E, Eimani H, Bigdeli MR, et al. Effects of crocin supplementation during in vitro maturation of mouse oocytes on glutathione synthesis and cytoplasmic maturation. International Journal of Fertility and Sterility. 2016;**10**(1):53-61

[20] Mokhber Maleki E, Eimani H, Bigdeli MR, et al. A comparative study of saffron aqueous extract and its active ingredient, crocin on the in vitro maturation, in vitro fertilization, and in vitro culture of mouse oocytes. Taiwanese Journal of Obstetrics & Gynecology. 2014;**53**(1):21-25

[21] Casillas F, Ducolomb Y, Lemus AE, et al. Porcine embryo production following in vitro fertilization and intracytoplasmic sperm injection from vitrified immature oocytes matured with a granulosa cell co-culture system. Cryobiology. 2015;**71**(2):299-305

[22] Abdel-Ghani MA, Shimizu T, Asano T, et al. In vitro maturation of canine oocytes co-cultured with bovine and canine granulosa cell monolayers. Theriogenology. 2012;**77**(2):347-355

[23] Choi BH, Bang JI, Jin JI, et al. Coculturing cumulus oocyte complexes with denuded oocytes alters zona pellucida ultrastructure in in vitro matured bovine oocytes. Theriogenology. 2013;**80**(9):1117-1123

[24] Shirazi A, Motaghi E. The in vitro fertilization of ovine oocytes in the presence of oviductal cells and its effect on the expression of zygote arrest 1 (Zar 1) and subsequent embryonic development. Journal of Reproduction & Infertility. 2013;**14**(1):8-16

[25] Ling B, Feng D-q, Zhou Y, et al. Effect of conditioned medium of mesenchymal stem cells on the in vitro maturation and subsequent development of mouse oocyte. Brazilian Journal of Medical and Biological Research. 2008;**41**(11):978-985

[26] Duarte Alcoba D, Gonsales Valrio E, Conzatti M, et al. Selection of developmentally competent human oocytes aspirated during cesarean section. The Journal of Maternal-Fetal & Neonatal Medicine. 2018;**31**(6):735-739

[27] Maman E, Meirow D, Brengauz M, et al. Luteal phase oocyte retrieval and in vitro maturation is an optional procedure for urgent fertility preservation. Fertility and Sterility. 2011;**95**(1):64-67

[28] Siristatidis C, Sergentanis TN, Vogiatzi P, et al. In vitro maturation in women with vs. without polycystic ovarian syndrome: A systematic review and meta-analysis. PLoS One. 2015;**10**(8):e0134696

[29] Reavey J, Vincent K, Child T, et al. Human chorionic gonadotrophin priming for fertility treatment with in vitro maturation. Cochrane Database of Systematic Reviews. 2016;**11**:CD008720

[30] Choavaratana R, Thanaboonyawat I, Laokirkkiat P, et al. Outcomes of follicle-stimulating hormone priming and nonpriming in in vitro maturation

of oocytes in infertile women with polycystic ovarian syndrome: A single-blinded randomized study. Gynecologic and Obstetric Investigation. 2015;**79**(3):153-159

[31] Fadini R, Dal Canto MB, Mignini Renzini M, et al. Effect of different gonadotrophin priming on IVM of oocytes from women with normal ovaries: A prospective randomized study. Reproductive Biomedicine Online. 2009;**19**(3):343-351

[32] Gilchrist RB. Recent insights into oocyte-follicle cell interactions provide opportunities for the development of new approaches to in vitro maturation. Reproduction, Fertility, and Development. 2011;**23**(1):23-31

[33] Swain JE. Optimal human embryo culture. Seminars in Reproductive Medicine. 2015;**33**(2):103-117

[34] Swain JE, Carrell D, Cobo A, et al. Optimizing the culture environment and embryo manipulation to help maintain embryo developmental potential. Fertility and Sterility. 2016;**105**(3):571-587

[35] Smith GD, Takayama S. Application of microfluidic technologies to human assisted reproduction. Molecular Human Reproduction. 2017;**23**(4):257-268

[36] Xiao S, Coppeta JR, Rogers HB, et al. A microfluidic culture model of the human reproductive tract and 28-day menstrual cycle. Nature Communications. 2017;**8**:14584

[37] Ledda S, Idda A, Kelly J, et al. A novel technique for in vitro maturation of sheep oocytes in a liquid marble microbioreactor. Journal of Assisted Reproduction and Genetics. 2016;**33**(4):513-518

[38] Omidi M, Khalili MA, Ashourzadeh S, et al. Zona pellucida birefringence and meiotic spindle visualisation of human oocytes are not influenced by IVM technology. Reproduction, Fertility, and Development. 2014;**26**(3):407-413

[39] Coticchio G, Dal Canto M, Fadini R, et al. Ultrastructure of human oocytes after in vitro maturation. Molecular Human Reproduction. 2016;**22**(2):110-118

[40] Dal Canto M, Novara PV, Coticchio G, et al. Morphokinetics of embryos developed from oocytes matured in vitro. Journal of Assisted Reproduction and Genetics. 2016;**33**(2):247-253

[41] Walls ML, Hart R, Keelan JA, et al. Structural and morphologic differences in human oocytes after in vitro maturation compared with standard in vitro fertilization. Fertility and Sterility. 2016;**106**(6):1392-1398

[42] Kuhtz J, Romero S, De Vos M, et al. Human in vitro oocyte maturation is not associated with increased imprinting error rates at LIT1, SNRPN, PEG3 and GTL2. Human Reproduction. 2014;**29**(9):1995-2005

[43] Yoshida H, Abe H, Arima T. Quality evaluation of IVM embryo and imprinting genes of IVM babies. Journal of Assisted Reproduction and Genetics. 2013;**30**(2):221-225

[44] Pliushch G, Schneider E, Schneider T, et al. In vitro maturation of oocytes is not associated with altered deoxyribonucleic acid methylation patterns in children from in vitro fertilization or intracytoplasmic sperm injection. Fertility and Sterility. 2015;**103**(3):720.e1-727.e1

[45] Chian RC, Xu CL, Huang JY, et al. Obstetric outcomes and congenital abnormalities in infants conceived with oocytes matured in vitro. Facts, Views & Vision in ObGyn. 2014;**6**(1):15-18

[46] Fadini R, Mignini Renzini M, Guarnieri T, et al. Comparison of the obstetric and perinatal outcomes of children conceived from in vitro or in vivo matured oocytes in in vitro maturation treatments with births from conventional ICSI cycles. Human Reproduction. 2012;**27**(12):3601-3608

[47] Chian RC, Uzelac PS, Nargund G. In vitro maturation of human immature oocytes for fertility preservation. Fertility and Sterility. 2013;**99**(5):1173-1181

Chapter 4

Oocyte Activation Failure: Physiological and Clinical Aspects

Nina Hojnik and Borut Kovačič

Abstract

Despite successful treatment of infertility with assisted reproductive technology (ART), total fertilization failure (TFF) after in vitro fertilization (IVF) and even after intracytoplasmic sperm injection (ICSI) still occurs. In the current chapter, the incidence and etiology of TFF after ICSI are described. The literature on physiology of oocyte activation, electrical properties of gametes' membranes, and ion currents is reviewed. Calcium oscillations play an essential role in fertilization, and calcium ions act as secondary messengers in different metabolic pathways and cellular processes during oocyte activation. The contribution of oocyte- and sperm-related causes of fertilization failure is discussed. Many studies on the physiology of fertilization in mammals have shown that oocyte activation is triggered by the sperm factor. Methods for artificial oocyte activation (AOA) try to bypass fertilization failure by influencing physiological processes that are crucial for successful fertilization. Activation can be induced with the use of electrical, mechanical, or chemical stimuli that elevate intracellular concentrations of calcium ions. Different AOA methods and their success and safety are presented.

Keywords: oocyte activation, total fertilization failure (TFF), calcium oscillations, artificial oocyte activation (AOA), gamete maturation, ion channels, ion currents, calcium signaling, meiosis, intracytoplasmic sperm injection (ICSI), PLCζ, calcium ionophores

1. Introduction

In vitro fertilization (IVF) techniques enabled conception outside the body and led to the birth of the first child conceived in vitro in 1978 [1]. The first laboratory technique used for conception in vitro was "classic" IVF where a suspension of prepared sperm cells is added to oocytes surrounded by cumulus cells and fertilization occurs naturally. The most discouraging result of such assisted reproduction technology (ART) treatment was fertilization failure, occurring often with the male infertility factor or unexplained infertility. The development of a micromanipulation technique named intracytoplasmic sperm injection (ICSI) in 1990 [2] enabled new treatment possibilities for many couples. Bypassing initial steps in the process of natural fertilization, a single spermatozoon is inserted directly into the cytoplasm. Successful fertilization is thus also achieved with low sperm numbers, surgically retrieved sperm, or frozen sperm samples. ICSI was soon globally accepted as a reliable technique leading to successful fertilization, pregnancy, and healthy offspring. Although ICSI can overcome some fertilization problems, total fertilization failure (TFF) still occurs in some ICSI cycles. In some patients, this failure can repeat in several ART cycles. Some patients have extremely low fertilization rates, which consequently lowers their chances for successful treatment.

Studies of etiology of fertilization failure after ICSI revealed that the predominant cause is oocyte activation failure [3, 4]. In humans, oocyte activation is the transition of the oocyte into a zygote where a series of intracellular calcium (Ca^{2+}) oscillations following the fusion of the gametes play an essential role. Calcium ions are released from intracellular storage in the endoplasmic reticulum; free in the cytosol, they are intracellular messengers and act as modulators of processes in the early steps of fertilization and embryo development. In humans, oocyte activation thus describes a cascade of events that lead to completion of the meiosis, cortical granule exocytosis for prevention of polyspermy, formation of the male and female pronuclei and progression in the first embryonic cell cycle. Both sperm and oocyte defects can cause failed activation.

Artificial oocyte activation (AOA) methods can be used in clinical practice in reproductive medicine in rare cases of TFF or low fertilization. AOA tries to reproduce elevations of calcium ion concentration in cytosol, which are necessary for triggering downstream processes in oocyte activation.

2. Total fertilization failure (TFF) after ICSI

Total fertilization failure after ICSI is complete lack of fertilization at the standard checking time of 17 ± 1 h post ICSI. This means that the obvious sign, female and male pronuclei, is not visible in any of the injected mature oocytes in the metaphase of meiosis II (MII) of the patient.

According to data from the literature, complete fertilization failure occurs in: 2 [5], 1.3 [6], 3 [7], 3 [8], 5.6 [9], and 4.3% [10] of ICSI cycles.

Complete fertilization failure after ICSI is directly correlated with the number of mature oocytes available [9], so the definition is needed. TFF is not surprising in cases of poor ovarian response, nonmotile spermatozoa, or poor sperm morphology. But even if we have a sufficient number of mature oocytes of normal morphology and sperm of good quality, TFF happens and can reoccur in subsequent cycles.

Another problem that also lowers the chances for successful treatment of infertility is an extremely low fertilization rate.

2.1 Results of retrospective analysis of data from our center

We analyzed all consecutive ICSI cycles in the period between years 2011 and 2016. Results are presented in **Table 1**. In this period, we performed 7474 ART cycles (IVF and ICSI) in our center. The majority of these cycles were stimulated with gonadotropins (recombinant FSH or highly purified human menopausal gonadotropin) with pituitary suppression using agonists or antagonists, followed by hCG administration for 36–37 h before ultrasound-guided follicle aspiration. Some of these cycles were natural cycles, as previously described in [11].

In this period, we performed 4533 ICSI cycles with at least one mature oocyte in the metaphase stage of meiosis II (MII) available. Complete fertilization failure (TFF) occurred in 247 (5.5%) of ICSI cycles.

We compared standard characteristics of these cycles regarding the number of oocytes. There were 3550 cycles with 3 or more MII oocytes, TFF occurred in 76 among the (2.14%) cycles. There were 983 cycles with 1 or 2 MII oocytes available, TFF occurred in 171 among them (17.4%). A total of 35 of these TFF cycles were natural cycles.

	Cycles with ≥3MII	Cycles with <3MII	Cycles with >0% and <30% fertilization (≥3MII)	Cycles with >70% fertilization (≥3MII)
N of all cycles	3550	983	175	1980
N of TFF cycles (%)	76 (2.14%)	171 (17.4%)	/	/
Woman age (years)	35.62 ± 4.42	37.26 ± 4.69	34.70 ± 4.96	34.14 ± 4.65
Stimulation protocol				
• Natural cycles	/	35 (20.5%)	/	/
• Long protocol with agonists GnRHa	26 (34.2%)	23 (13.5%)	58 (33.1%)	595 (30.6%)
• Short protocol with antagonists antGnRH	45 (59.2%)	101 (59.1%)	105 (60.0%)	1297 (65.1%)
• Other	5	12	12	88
Duration of stimulation	10.40 ± 1.95	8.77 ± 4.85	9.96 ± 1.76	9.98 ± 1.8
Gonadotropin dose (ampoules)	32.80 ± 11.84	31.53 ± 20.72	28.86 ± 10.75	27.34 ± 9.92
N oocytes	8.04 ± 6.10	2.02 ± 2.46	10.16 ± 5.4	10.16 ± 5.95
MII	5.80 ± 4.13	1.25 ± 0.44	7.91 ± 4.41	8.51 ± 5.07
2PN	0	0	1.35 ± 1.21	7.37 ± 4.33
1PN	0.07 ± 0.25	0.09 ±0.30	0.16 ± 0.40	0.12 ± 0.37
3PN	0.16 ± 0.49	0.26 ± 1.11	0.22 ± 0.64	0.10 ± 0.35
Damaged	0.29 ± 0.82	0.26 ± 1.11	0.57 ± 1.06	0.22 ± 0.55
Male diagnosis				
• Normozoospermia (% of TFF cycles)	15 (19.74%)	61 (35.67%)	31 (17.7%)	371 (18.7%)
• Krypto- and azoospermia (% of TFF cycles)	18 (23.68%)	17 (9.94%)	45 (25.7%)	214 (10.8%)
ET	0	0	1.04 ± 0.76	1.57 ± 0.69
Clinical pregnancy	/	/	39/220 17.7%	702/1822 38.5%
Birth rate	/	/	13.2%	30.5%

Table 1.
Analysis of all consecutive ICSI cycles performed in our clinic in the period between years 2011 and 2016 (N = 4533); cycles with at least one mature oocyte in the metaphase stage of meiosis II (MII) are included. Data are presented in means ± SD or number of cases (percentage of all cases in a group).

We also analyzed the characteristics of cycles with 3 or more MII oocytes and low fertilization; in doing so, we took into account cycles with more than 0% and less than 30% MII oocytes fertilized. There were 175 such cycles (3.9%).

Woman's age is greater in cycles with fewer oocytes, which can be explained with lower ovarian reserve in greater age. Regarding the stimulation protocol of the ART cycles, there were 35 natural cycles in the group with <3 MII oocytes. In our center, natural cycles are mainly performed in patients with extremely low ovarian response, where increasing gonadotropin dosage does not increase the chance to obtain more oocytes.

In TFF cases where 3 or more MII oocytes are available, there is a higher proportion of severe male infertility cases (22.68%) compared to the cycles with less than

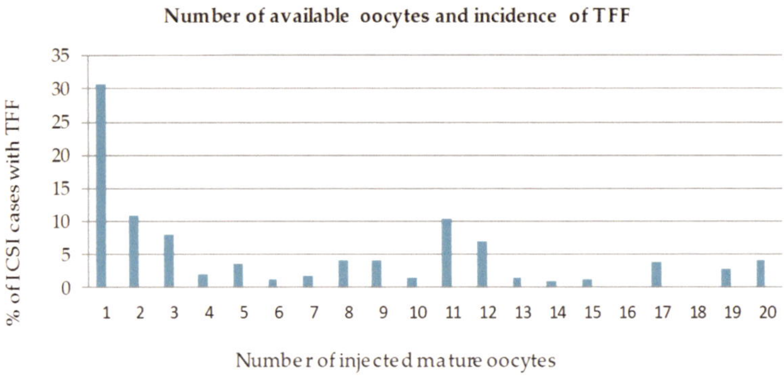

Figure 1.
Number of available oocytes and incidence of TFF. The proportion of ICSI cycles with total fertilization failure regarding the number of mature oocytes available; x = number of injected MII oocytes; y = % of cycles with TFF. 4533 ICSI cycles analysed.

3 MII oocytes (9.94%). When there are more oocytes available, there is statistically less probability for TFF, and more cases of TFF are due to gamete defects. A similar proportion of low fertilization cycles are those with severe male infertility (25.7%). Severe male infertility is described as diagnosis of cryptozoospermia and azoospermia, where individual sperms have to be extracted from semen sediments or testis aspirates/biopsies.

In cases where only one mature oocyte was available, total fertilization failure occurred more often (30.8%) than in those with more oocytes.

In **Figure 1**, the correlation between the number of available mature oocytes and occurrence of TFF is presented. With more oocytes available, there is less probability for TFF.

3. Etiology of failed fertilization after ICSI

Soon after implementation of the ICSI technique, some investigations of possible reasons for unsuccessful fertilization began. It was first speculated that perhaps the proportion of unfertilized oocytes arises from technical limitations of the method itself that cannot deliver the sperm in the cytoplasm, or ejection of the sperm from the cytoplasm occurs after injection. It was established that in only 7 [12], 16.7 [7], 10.6 [13], and 12.6% [14] of unfertilized oocytes after ICSI the sperm DNA was outside the oocytes.

With different staining techniques, visualization of the chromatin, spindle, and other structures was possible, and this enabled a better understanding of at what stage unfertilized oocytes are (**Table 2**). It soon became evident that the majority of unfertilized oocytes are arrested in the metaphase of the meiosis II with different levels of sperm chromatin decondensation, which suggested that oocyte activation and sperm decondensation run independently [15]. In the majority of these oocytes, sperm chromatin is in a decondensed state, which indicates that protamines are usually successfully replaced by histones [14], so unsuccessful decondensation of sperm chromatin can be the underlying cause for only a relatively small proportion of unfertilized oocytes. Premature chromosome condensation (PCC) is a condition when sperm chromosomes are getting condensed in the cytoplasm of oocyte too early and the right synchronization between sperm and oocyte genetic material is compromised. Up to 33% of studied unfertilized oocytes had PCC [15], but it is difficult to conclude whether this indicates sperm- or oocyte-borne defect.

The studies are summarized in **Table 2**.

Study	Method	Number of analyzed specimens	Findings
Flaherty SP, Payne D, and Matthews CD [7]	Hoechst 33342: fluorescent stain for adenine-thymine rich regions in DNA	n = 1005 NF MII	82% of oocytes are arrested in metaphase MII; of these, 74% decondensed SC, 11% intact SC, 15% without sperm in the cytoplasm
			only 17% of oocytes activated; of these 56% decondensed SC, 20% intact SC, 15% without sperm in the cytoplasm
Dozortsev D, Sutter PD, and Dhont M [12]	Giemsa: stain for adenine-thymine rich regions in DNA	n = 82 NF MII	93% oocytes having sperm in cytoplasm and MII chromosomes of the oocyte present; of these 51% SC, 41% intact SC, 8% premature chromosome condensation (PCC)
Yanagida K [13]	Aceto-orcein stain: chromatin staining	n = 76 NF MII	86.8% oocytes having sperm in cytoplasm; of these 68.2% decondensed SC, 4.5% PCC, 27.3% intact SC
Pitsos MA, Nicolopoulou-Stamati P [14]	Chromomycin A3: binds to G-C rich DNA regions, does not bind to DNA coupled with protamines Propidium iodide: fluorescent DNA stain	n = 93 NF MII	74.8% metaphase MII oocytes; of these 63.6% decondensed SC, 23.4% condensed SC, and 13% no sperm in the cytoplasm. In majority of spermatozoa, successful replacement of protamines with histones took place.
Rawe VY, Olmedo SB, Nodar FN, Doncel GD, Acosta AA, and Vitullo AD [16]	Immunofluorescence analysis with immunoglobulins and monoclonal antibodies	n = 150 NF MII	13.3% oocytes with no sperm, 39.9% activation failure, 22.6% defects of pronuclear formation/migration, 13.3% arrest in metaphase of the 1st mitotic division
Kovacic B and Vlaisavljevic V [15]	Hoechst 33258, FITC	n = 180 NF MII	69% oocytes arrested in metaphase MII, 11% completed meiosis, but no PN development

SC = sperm chromatin, MII = mature oocyte in metaphase of meiosis II, NF = non-fertilized oocyte, and PCC = premature chromosome condensation.

Table 2.
Studies of the etiology of fertilization failure.

On the basis of the studies listed in **Table 2**, we can conclude that failed oocyte activation seems to be the predominant reason for fertilization failure. However, it is unclear whether the cause is sperm or oocyte defect, since proteins, organelles, and metabolic paths of both gametes are involved in the activation.

Oocyte activation failure being the main problem was also confirmed by electron microscopy, where unreleased cortical granule at periphery, maternal chromosomes in the metaphase plate, and paternal intact or partially decondensed chromatin were found [3]. These are all signs of failed activation, but it is difficult to conclude on which level in the cascade there is a failure.

Perhaps, in the future, genetic data will give us more information on the etiology of fertilization failure. An interesting case report where researchers investigated possible reasons for fertilization failure on genetic levels analyzed gene expression profiles in unfertilized oocytes of a patient with previous TFF history [17].

4. Oocyte activation

Oocyte activation is a downstream cascade triggered by sperm that causes progression of the oocyte from meiosis arrested in metaphase II toward its completion and beginning of embryonic development. It is a serial of biochemical reactions, organelle redistribution, changes in metabolism, transmembrane potentials, mRNA translation, gene transcription, and cytoskeletal rearrangements.

The role of calcium in fertilization was established very early with a series of experiments on sea urchin eggs where the amount of bound and free calcium was measured in fertilized and nonfertilized eggs [18]. Later, calcium-specific light-emitting protein aequorin injected in fish oocytes enabled visualization of light flash after fusion of oocyte and sperm [19]. It soon became evident that calcium ions play an essential role in activation of the animal oocyte and that the frequencies and amplitudes of these elevations of calcium ions in cytoplasm are species-specific [20].

The term "oocyte activation" probably evolved on the basis of these evident sudden changes that happen during the transition from oocyte to embryo. It describes not only calcium waves that occur but also other processes and morphological changes that happen during fertilization. Intracytoplasmic calcium elevation is essential for fertilization, but it is not always the sperm that triggers it. In some animal species such as fruit flies (*Drosophila*) the calcium wave occurs prior to oocyte-sperm fusion, during ovulation [21]. The focus of our text will be human oocyte activation, but since nonhuman biological material is usually more available or even easier to study, many data on fertilization come from studies on sea organisms such as starfish and sea urchins or different mammalian species. Early studies of the role of calcium in the process of fertilization and even use of ionophores are well documented in the review of Epel [22]. The source of an intracellular rise of calcium ion concentration can be external—calcium enters the cell by influx through calcium channels in the plasma membrane or can be released in cytoplasm from intracellular stores in the endoplasmic reticulum [23].

But it is important to understand that the details vary a lot through the animal kingdom and that these differences can be the reason why the ICSI method can be successful in humans but not in other species. However, the animal studies are the foundation for the development of assisted reproduction techniques in human medicine.

Early studies of fertilization in mammals are well reviewed by Miyazaki [24]; in sum, there is the first hyperpolarization of membrane potential as a result of a change in potassium conductivity across the plasma membrane. This coincides with an increase of free calcium in cytosol; there is no electrical block of polyspermy and a serial of intracytoplasmic rises of calcium concentration follow continuously (oscillations) at intervals of different frequencies and amplitudes, which depends on the species studied. Intracellular calcium first rises near the site of the sperm attachment and spreads like a wave over the entire egg [24]. The model of generating calcium spikes from intracellular stores in the endoplasmic reticulum was described by Igusa and Miyazaki [25]. The techniques used for revealing these processes were measurements with calcium-sensitive microelectrodes, the voltage-clamp technique, aequorin injections, injection of calcium ion chelators, and injection of different compounds that interact with the calcium-releasing system.

The first study of calcium measurements at fertilization in human oocytes showed that the first rise in intracytoplasmic calcium concentration appears 20–35 min after adding sperm suspension in a chamber with oocytes; spikes appear every 10–35 min, with a single spike of amplitude up to 2.25 μM calcium concentration and duration of 100–120 s [26].

Other researchers studied changes of membrane potential across the plasma membrane in human oocytes at fertilization and showed that the increase of potassium ion conductivity of the plasma membrane and outward current of ions, which causes hyperpolarization, is calcium dependent [27]. A study on bovine oocytes gave more information about the relationship between hyperpolarization of the plasma membrane potential and calcium release from intracellular stores and targeted calcium-activated potassium channels as membrane proteins involved in the process [28].

Soon after introducing ICSI, it was of great interest to compare these responses with the classic IVF method, where events such as sperm capacitation and activation, acrosome reaction, and sperm-oocyte membrane fusion happen first. From the work of Tesarik et al. [29], we can see that when performing ICSI in human oocytes, the first intracytoplasmic rise of calcium ion concentration happens immediately; the peak is 10–15 s after penetration with the needle. Sperm then evokes intracellular calcium oscillations. They described that oscillations follow the lag period that lasts 4–12 h. Oscillations are in the form of spikes that last 20 s; the intervals between spikes are 1–5 min. The duration of the oscillatory phase is 30 min–1 h; at the end of the period, the amplitude of calcium spikes gets smaller.

The proposed mechanism through which calcium oscillations are maintained is through the phosphoinositide signaling pathway, where inositol 1,4,5-trisphosphate ($InsP_3$) is generated from phosphatidylinositol 4,5-bisphosphate (PIP_2) [23]. The positive feedback cycle involving calcium-dependent $InsP_3$ generation and $InsP_3$-induced calcium release seem to be responsible for the oscillations [23]. The main protein is $InsP_3$ receptor ($InsP_3R$), a ligand-gated channel found in the membrane of the endoplasmic reticulum that allows calcium release from the ER [30].

That calcium oscillations have a role in long-term embryonic events and provide more than merely a stimulus for meiotic resumption was shown in experiments with different activating agents and subsequent measurements of cell mass of the blastocyst [31].

4.1 The role of free calcium ions in cytoplasm

Calcium is the secondary messenger that regulates different events during fertilization, such as progression of the cell cycle from metaphase II arrest toward chromatid segregation, extrusion of the second polar body and completion of the second meiotic division, and cortical granule exocytosis [32]. The role of calcium in reproduction is preserved through evolution; it is important in plants and animals. Species-specific calcium signatures, like oscillations in mammals, have evolved, which are optimal for activation and development of a specific type of organism [33]. The variations in amplitude, duration, and frequency of oscillations over time are coordinated with the cell cycle, and experimentally changing them also affects development in the later stages when blastocyst forms [31]. Experiments with injecting calcium (Ca^{2+}) chelators in the cytosol of frog eggs demonstrated the blockage of activation [34].

Calcium rises in cytosol are converted in different cellular responses.

4.1.1 Ca^{2+}-dependent process of cortical granule exocytosis

Cortical granule exocytosis enables polyspermy block by altering the zona pellucida with the content of the granule (proteases, peroxidases, and glycosaminoglycans) and prevent more sperms from fertilizing oocytes. The proposed model is that calcium stimulates Ca^{2+}/calmodulin (CaM)-dependent protein kinase

II (CaMKII) and myosin light-chain kinase (MLCK) that phosphorylate a vesicle targeting protein and myosin II to promote exocytosis [33]. It is a quick response; in mouse oocytes, exocytosis starts 15 min after exposure to capacitated sperm, and 30 min after insemination, 78% of cortical granules disappear from cytoplasm [35]. It is proposed that each calcium oscillation cycle moves cortical granule one step closer to the egg plasma membrane toward the fusion with the plasma membrane and exocytosis of the contents [33].

4.1.2 Ca^{2+} is a trigger for cell cycle progression

The completion of meiosis means that the extrusion of the chromatids in the second polar body enables the formation of haploid oocytes that can form a female pronucleus that will be able to combine genetic material with the male pronucleus.

Meiosis is the ground of sexual reproduction where homologous chromosomes recombine—exchange genetic material through chiasmata and generate new genetic combinations that are unique to the offspring. Mammalian oocytes progress through meiosis very slowly; first, the cell cycle is arrested in the dictyate phase of prophase I during the fetal life of a girl and stays in this phase up to 40–50 years. During the menstrual cycle, the recruited oocytes in the ovary progress through the cell cycle under the influence of the hormones. But the meiosis is again arrested at the metaphase of the second meiotic division (metMII). Calcium oscillations at fertilization activate calmodulin-dependent protein kinase II (CaMKII) and switch on the anaphase-promoting complex/cyclosome (APC/C) that leads to securin and cyclin B1 degradation necessary for cell cycle progression and segregation of sister chromatids [33].

Ca^{2+} also plays a role in pronuclear formation by decreasing MAP kinase (MAPK) activity responsible for nuclear envelope assembly [33]. Oscillations terminate with PN formation, and PLCζ localizes into PN [36]. The mechanism by which Ca^{2+} recruits maternal mRNA for translation and genome activation is not well understood at the moment. There are some data indicating that calcium oscillations and mRNA translation are coupled [37]. Not only in cytosol, calcium can also diffuse to the nucleus and control different cell functions by direct nuclear calcium signaling [38].

4.2 Electrophysiology and fertilization

Fertilization potential is a change in the membrane potential across the plasma membrane (PM) of the oocyte that is first observed after oocyte-sperm interaction. In many invertebrates, this is in the form of depolarization of the plasma membrane and is proposed to provide a fast block to polyspermy, described in some invertebrates and only a few vertebrates (such as frogs), but not present in mammals [39]. Lately, there have been some discussions about the nature of electrical block in preventing polyspermy [40]. The role of electrical events in the form of depolarization or hyperpolarization of the plasma membrane at fertilization remains unclear.

In mammals, there is hyperpolarization of membrane potential as a result of change in potassium conductivity across the plasma membrane [24]. In human oocytes, outward current and long-lasting hyperpolarization of the plasma membrane were described [27]. The channels responsible for this hyperpolarization are calcium-activated potassium channels [41]. Species-specific differences in the channels involved in early electrical responses at fertilization are reviewed in [42].

During oocyte maturation, the composition of the channels in the plasma membrane changes, as described in bovine oocytes [28]. The factors regulating the composition of channels in the plasma membrane, the conductance for different ions, depending on the specificity, gating, and sensitivity of the channels at different stages, are still unclear. The conditions during gamete maturation are very important, and we can imagine that diet and changes in metabolic pathways can affect the performance. It is not just cytoplasmic maturity of the oocyte that is important, but also maturity of the plasma membrane.

The conditions in which gametes are matured are important; the diet and especially taking some medicines in this period can affect the infertility treatment outcome. There are some data from studies of calcium channel blockers used as therapy in various cardiovascular conditions. They affect the movement of free calcium ions across membranes, and dose-dependent reduction in sperm mobility and viability in vitro that can affect fertility treatment was demonstrated [43].

4.3 Sperm factors

Data from studies of fertilization pointed to a sperm component that has to trigger response in the form of calcium oscillations. But the exact component, its nature, and mechanism were long unknown.

There were four main hypotheses, reviewed in [44]. The first one assumed that sperm delivers calcium to the oocyte that further stimulates release of calcium from intracellular stores. The conduit hypothesis assumed that sperm increases the permeability of the plasma membrane for calcium that enters the oocyte with influx from the surroundings. The contact hypothesis predicts that sperm interacts with a receptor on the plasma membrane that causes calcium release from intracellular stores. But success of the ICSI method revealed that there is no need for interaction of sperm and receptors in the plasma membrane for fertilization. The fourth is the sperm factor hypothesis that assumes that there is a component in the sperm cell delivered in cytosol with sperm and that this factor causes calcium release from intracellular stores.

Experiments where soluble sperm extracts are injected into the oocyte coupled with different biochemical approaches enabled the search for unknown sperm factor and were in favor of the sperm factor hypothesis [45, 46].

There were many candidates such as oscillin, a cytosolic sperm factor related to prokaryote glucosamine phosphate deaminase [47]. In nonmammalian species, PLCγ was identified [48] and the role of nitric oxide in fertilization was investigated [49]. In mammals post-acrosomal WW domain-binding protein (PAWP) was described, which is located in the post-acrosomal region of the sperm, from the stage of elongated spermatids onwards, that causes meiosis resumption and PN formation [50].

4.3.1 PLCζ

When it was demonstrated that sperm extracts were related to $InsP_3$ concentrations in cell and PLC activity [51], phospholipases were under investigation. Genetic data from the testis' cDNA library revealed some new isoform of PLC [23] and soon a novel sperm-specific phospholipase C, PLCζ was identified as a trigger of calcium oscillations in mouse eggs [52]. In the work of Saunders et al., it was experimentally demonstrated that PLCζ content in a single sperm evoked oscillations and normal embryonic development [52]. They also prepared PLCζ complementary RNA (cRNA) for injection into MII oocytes that triggered the same effect. When they removed PLCζ from sperm extracts, they no longer induced calcium oscillations.

Important evidence that PLCζ is the necessary trigger for calcium oscillations comes also from the studies of Dpy19l2 knockout mice that have globozoospermic sperm phenotype and absence of or extremely reduced PLC ζ and no ability to trigger calcium oscillations [53]. But proof in the form of the knockout mouse model was missing. By using RNA interference technology that prevents translation of PLCζ mRNA and that reduces the amount of PLCζ protein in transgenic mouse sperm, altered calcium oscillation patterns, lower egg activation, and no transgenic offspring [54] were observed.

A study where whole exome sequencing was performed in patients with previous TFF, homozygous missense mutation in PLCζ was established [55].

PLCζ was identified in many mammalian and nonmammalian species [56, 57] and can act across species. But there are differences in solubility of PLCζ in cytosol that can contribute to differences between species. It is proven in the mouse oocyte activation test (MOAT) that human PLCζ exhibits greater response in mouse oocytes than mouse PLCζ.

The amount of PLCζ measured in a single mouse sperm cell is in the same range as the amount required to cause oscillations experimentally [52]. This can explain why altered frequency of oscillations was established when more than one sperm fertilized an oocyte [58]. PLCζ has to diffuse through cytosol to trigger spatiotemporal response in the form of a calcium wave that spreads from the point of sperm entry to the other pole.

Recently, the knockout mouse model was prepared using CRISPR/Cas9 gene editing [59] and revealed interesting facts: PLCζ-null mouse males have normal spermatogenesis and normal sperm parameters (motility, capacitation, and acrosome reaction) but their sperm cannot elicit calcium oscillations after ICSI. Still, some oocytes can undergo activation in abnormal form or even develop to blastocyst stage. But mating knockout males with normal females shows that they can still produce offspring without PLCζ as a physiological trigger. Males are not infertile, rather subfertile, so there is possibility that apart from PLCζ, there is a second calcium releasing factor delivered to oocyte by sperm, perhaps an alternative that is used only when PLCζ is missing.

Calcium oscillations are normal physiological stimuli for oocyte activation but from parthenogenetic activation at ICSI and from the use of artificial oocyte activation techniques we already know that they are not always necessary to activate oocytes. They can be bypassed on some levels.

There are still many facts about calcium oscillations triggering that are not well understood. The proposed mechanism of activation is reviewed in [23] and represented in a schematic diagram (**Figure 2**): PLCζ diffuses from the sperm head into egg cytosol and hydrolyses the PIP_2 (phosphatidylinositol 4,5-bisphosphate) in the membrane of the vesicle compartment into products $InsP_3$ (inositol 1,4,5-trisphosphate) and DAG (diacylglycerol). $InsP_3$ binds to the receptor $InsP_3R$ on the endoplasmic reticulum membrane. The conformation of the channel is changed and it becomes permeable for Ca^{2+} ions that are released from intracellular storage in the endoplasmic reticulum into cytosol. Oscillations are generated through a positive feedback loop.

In a series of experiments on mouse oocytes injected with RNA encoding PLCζ and tagged with a fluorescent protein, it was established that at the time when calcium oscillations terminate and pronucleus is formed, PLCζ protein translocates from the cytosol to the pronucleus [36]. Authors also demonstrated that it is again released in the cytosol in the first mitotic division of an embryo at the time of nuclear envelope breakdown and observed also in the second mitotic division. This suggests the possible role of calcium oscillations not only in oocyte activation but also in early embryonic development.

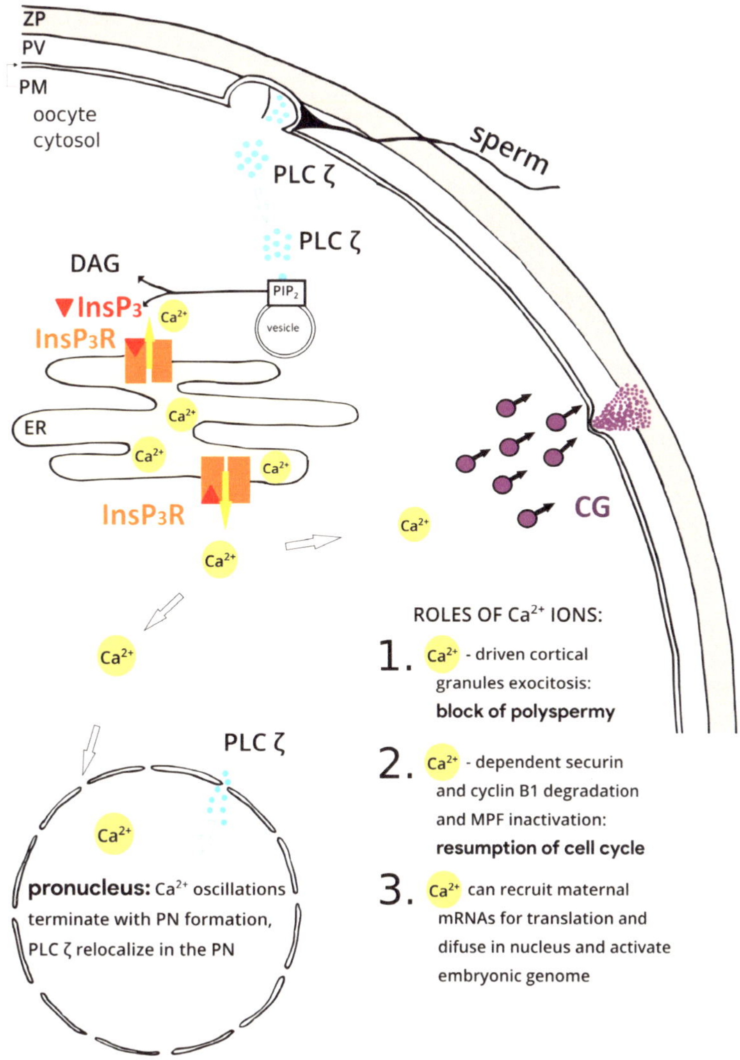

Figure 2.
Schematic diagram of the proposed model of sperm triggered oocyte activation at fertilization in mammals: after the fusion of sperm and oocyte plasma membrane PLCζ diffuses from sperm into oocyte cytosol. Vesicles baring PIP_2 are present in cytosol and PLCζ hydrolyzes PIP_2 into products DAG and $InsP_3$. $InsP_3$ binds to the $InsP_3R$ present in the membrane of ER. $InsP_3R$ is a ligand-gated Ca^{2+} release channel and Ca^{2+} is released from intracellular stores in ER into the cytosol. In mammals, repetitive Ca^{2+} oscillations occur, and several rises of calcium concentration in cytosol take place. Ca^{2+} ions play an essential role in oocyte activation. They enable block of polyspermy by chemically altering zona pellucida with the content of cortical granules that are released in the perivitelline space. Ca^{2+} ions enable cell cycle progression—resumption of meiosis II. Ca^{2+}-dependent inactivation of factors that hold cell cycle in arrested state takes place, by degradation of cyclinB1 and securin and MPF inactivation of cell cycle eventually progresses. Ca^{2+} ions play a role in recruitment of mRNAs and affect their translation. Ca^{2+} can diffuse in the nucleus and play a role in embryonic gene activation. Ca^{2+} oscillations terminate when female pronucleus is formed and PLCζ relocalizes in the pronucleus. PLCζ—phospholipase C zeta, PIP_2—phosphatidylinositol 4,5-bisphosphate, $InsP_3$—inositol 1,4,5-trisphosphate, DAG—diacylglycerol, $InsP_3R$—inositol 1,4,5-trisphosphate receptor, Ca^{2+}—calcium ions, ZP—zona pellucida (the glycoprotein envelope surrounding mammalian oocyte), PV—perivitelline space (space between ZP and plasma membrane of oocyte), PM—plasma membrane, cg—cortical granules, and PN—pronucleus.

All together there is a lot of accumulating evidence that points toward PLCζ as a trigger of oocyte activation cascade in mammals. Soon the idea of using recombinant PLCζ in clinical practice emerged that will be discussed later among other methods for artificial oocyte activation. But still there are many data missing that are needed to fully understand oocyte activation.

4.3.2 Other sperm-related factors that affect oocyte activation

Spermatozoon has to go through many changes in order to be able to fertilize an oocyte naturally. First, the mechanism of chemotaxis between the gametes plays an important role; capacitation is the process of altering the sperm plasma membrane so that it becomes more permanent for calcium ions, then changes in sperm movements in the form of hyperactivation help to bring the spermatozoon closer to the oocyte. Finally, at acrosome reaction the content of acrosomes (enzymes) facilitates the fusion between the plasma membrane of the oocyte and spermatozoon so that the paternal genetic material can enter the oocyte. Sperm also delivers a centriole into the oocyte that duplicates and forms centrosome, a microtubule-organizing center responsible for mitotic divisions in a growing embryo. ICSI bypasses many of these events and enables fertilization and successful development, but there are still sperm factors other than PLCζ that can contribute to failure of oocyte activation.

Successful sperm chromatin decondensation is a necessary condition for fertilization. The chromatin of the spermatozoon is uniquely packaged in such a way that histones become replaced by protamines during the spermatogenesis. Protamines provide more structural stability but after the entry of the spermatozoon into the oocyte the chromatin of the spermatozoon must be uncoiled and protamines must be replaced by histones. Proteins and other factors in the cytosol of an oocyte play a role in the correct decondensation of male genetic material.

Mitosis-promoting factor (MPF) in the cytosol of an oocyte can cause premature chromosome condensation (PCC), but perhaps it is not only an oocyte-related problem. It was established that protamine-deficient sperm seems to be related to a higher proportion of PCC independent of oocyte cytoplasmic maturity [60, 61]. The cell cycle of spermatozoa is related to chromatin status and protamine-histone remodeling must be synchronized with the oocyte.

4.4 Oocyte factors

If PLCζ depletion in sperm is a good candidate for explaining fertilization failure of male origin, less is known about different oocyte defects that cause unsuccessful activation. It is obvious that oocyte maturation is crucial and competent oocytes of good quality with all the necessary elements in the downstream cascade must be available. In the process of oocyte maturation, not only the elements responsible for generating calcium oscillations must develop but also all other elements such as those responsible for exocytosis of cortical granules, the necessary actin cortical cytoskeleton, and energy resources must be available.

The direct proof of oocyte-borne defects is the results of the mouse oocyte activation test (MOAT) that will be discussed in detail later. It is a heterologous model where mouse oocytes are fertilized with the patient's sperm. Successful fertilization of mouse oocytes points toward oocyte defects that are the underlying cause of previous fertilization failure in ART treatments in a specific couple.

4.4.1 Organelle distribution

Studies of the ultrastructure of unfertilized oocytes with transmission or scanning electron microscopy revealed differences in oocyte ultrastructure that can reflect different stages in oocyte maturation [62].

Cortical granule migration toward the plasma membrane is an important step in cytoplasmic maturation and it is a cytoskeleton-dependent process [63].

Some studies have investigated the relationship between mitochondrial function and fertilization. Unfertilized oocytes exhibit a higher proportion of mtDNA deletions that may contribute to their malfunction and ATP production [64]. As the early embryo requires a lot of energy, it is important that during oocyte maturation a sufficient number and functionality of the mitochondria are prepared.

Reorganization of the endoplasmic reticulum (ER) during maturation seems to play an important role in oocyte competence to generate calcium oscillations. Visualization of the ER in mouse oocytes revealed that in prophase I (in the germinal vesicle stage) the ER is in the form of a fine network with patch-like accumulations in the inner cytoplasm. After the resumption of meiosis, the ER accumulates in the form of a dense ring in the center of the oocyte, around the meiotic apparatus; later the ER rings move together with a meiotic spindle toward the oocyte cortex [65]. In oocytes in metaphase II, the ER ring transforms into clusters in the cortical region; in the central cytoplasm the reticular form is present [65]. These researchers also showed that these relocalizations happen independently from meiotic progression and that microtubules, dyneins, and actins are responsible for the movements.

During oocyte maturation, the Ins_3R receptors responsible for calcium release from the endoplasmic reticulum achieve their functionality. In a mouse model, it was demonstrated that increase in IP_3R1 sensitivity is underpinned, at least in part, by increases in calcium concentrations within the endoplasmic reticulum and receptor phosphorylation but not by changes in IP_3R1 distribution [66].

Distribution of vesicles with PIP_2 is also important. PLCζ diffuses from the sperm head into egg cytosol and acts on PIP_2 that is present in the membrane of small vesicles in the cytoplasm. Defects or deficits of PIP_2 or vesicles could contribute to fertilization failure [30].

4.4.2 Cytoplasmic maturation

Evaluation of oocyte maturity relies on the presence of the first polar body, but it is difficult to evaluate in daily IVF laboratory practice whether the oocyte cytoplasm is mature.

Cytoplasmic maturity is an important factor determining the ability of the oocyte to activate. During oocyte cytoplasmic maturation, the mechanisms responsible for sperm-induced calcium oscillations and oocyte activation develop and are reviewed in [67].

It was experimentally shown in LT/Sv mouse strain (that has abnormal oocyte nuclear maturation arrested at metaphase I) that the ability of these oocytes to be activated by sperm develops gradually during cytoplasmic maturation independent of nuclear maturation [68].

Oocyte cytoplasmic maturity also plays a role in decondensation of the sperm genetic material that is tightly packed with protamines. Oocyte immaturity is correlated to the occurrence of premature chromosome condensation (PCC) of the male pronucleus [69].

Evaluation of cytoplasmic maturity with immunocytochemical methods revealed that metaphase plate rearrangements are more frequent in oocytes showing immaturity [70]. Another study investigated abnormal maturation in patients with a high proportion of immature oocytes [71].

It is obvious that the conditions in which oocytes mature are important and beside patient-related factors there are also cycle-specific factors that have an impact on oocyte maturity, quality, and fertilization. Little is known about the cellular mechanisms of how diet, medicament uptake, or tobacco/alcohol intake affect oocyte quality. In a review of [72], the environmental impact on oocyte function through mitochondrial level is discussed.

5. Artificial oocyte activation (AOA)

Artificial oocyte activation methods try to induce oocyte activation by using physiological properties of the gametes and in this way interfere in different levels of the cascade of events during fertilization. In general, they try to alleviate intracellular calcium concentration and mimic oscillations. As we are well aware by now that there is big species-specific variability in the mechanisms of oocyte activation, it is not surprising that different AOA methods can be successful in one species, but not in another.

By influencing gamete physiological properties such as electrical excitability and plasma membrane conductivity, the aim is to increase intracytoplasmic calcium concentrations and mimic the frequency and amplitude of the oscillations.

Basically, there are three types of AOA methods: electrical, chemical, and mechanical.

5.1 Electrical methods

By applying direct electrical current within a Petri dish with oocytes, the electrical field stimulates charged proteins to move toward the plasma membrane, and by this, the number of pores in the plasma membrane increases [30]. Calcium conductivity increases, and more calcium enters the oocyte from the surroundings. There is only one large calcium concentration increase.

In the prospective randomized study of [73], an electrical pulse in a special chamber with electrodes 30 minutes after ICSI in 0.3 M glucose drops was used to activate oocytes, and a small increase in the fertilization rate after ICSI was achieved. Successful pregnancy and birth were achieved and reported in the case report [74].

In a study with round spermatid injection coupled with electrostimulation, the electrical pulse triggered not only a single calcium concentration increase, but a series of calcium spikes after spermatid injection [75].

5.2 Chemical methods

Chemical activation is the most commonly used method. Oocytes are exposed to chemical agents that lead to an increase in intracellular calcium concentration in the oocyte. Some agents, such as calcium ionophores cause a single, prolonged calcium transient, while others cause multiple oscillations.

5.2.1 Ionophores

Calcium ionophores, such as ionomycin, A23187 (calcimycin), and gm508 are molecules soluble in lipids, synthesized by microorganisms; today several synthetic compounds are known. They can transport ions across lipid bilayers. They increase membrane permeability for Ca^{2+} ions, thus allowing calcium influx in the oocyte from the surrounding medium and intracytoplasmic rise of calcium concentration. It has been recently established that intracytoplasmic rise of calcium concentration in human and mouse oocytes is not only the consequence of the influx from the surroundings but also from intracellular stores, since this rise appears also in calcium-free medium. However, they are not able to induce calcium oscillations typical for mammalian species but a single rise. Different protocols are described in the literature, regarding different concentrations used, and intervals of ionophore exposition [76–79].

They are used in cases of repeating TFF or low fertilization, oligoteratoasthenospermia cases, globozoospermia, in vitro maturation of oocytes (IVM), unexplained female infertility, and low ovarian reserve, with patients with Kartagener's syndrome with no response on theophylline, at primary ciliary dyskinesia. They are the most widely used chemical agents for artificial oocyte activation.

5.2.2 Strontium chloride ($SrCl_2$)

It is reported as very efficient in mice and induces not only single calcium concentration elevation, but oscillations [80]. The mechanism by which it induces oscillations is not fully understood.

A study that investigated efficacy of $SrCl_2$ in human oocytes showed significantly increased fertilization rates, when compared with conventional ICSI or calcium ionophore treatment [81].

5.2.3 PLCζ

Soon after the discovery of the role of PLCζ as a trigger of oocyte activation, the ideas of using the protein as an artificial activator emerged. The synthesis of the first recombinant human PLCζ protein was published [82]; when injected into mouse oocytes, calcium oscillations were evoked that closely resembled those initiated by the sperm after fertilization. Later, a study where human recombinant PLCζ was used on human and mouse oocytes was published [83] describing dose-dependent manner of calcium oscillations. These authors also showed that by injecting recombinant human PLCζ the next day in oocytes that failed to fertilize after ICSI, five of eight oocytes were rescued.

Earlier, it was established that PLCζ complementary RNA (cRNA) injection in MII oocytes also triggered oscillations [52] with a time lag that enables protein to synthesize.

The commercial use of recombinant human PLCζ still has to be validated in terms of safety.

5.2.4 Ethanol

In veterinary medicine, ethanol is often used for parthenogenetic oocyte activation. Parthenogenesis is development of an embryo from an unfertilized oocyte, naturally occurring in invertebrates or even some vertebrates. By inhibiting the second polar body extrusion, diploid parthenotes with two maternal genomes can be created and embryos can develop normally for several days, but later die. In several species, artificial parthenogenetic activation was described to be caused by ethanol [84].

5.3 Mechanical methods

Some data from the literature suggest that the modified ICSI technique can give better fertilization in patients with a history of TFF or low fertilization [85, 86]. Vigorous aspiration of cytoplasm and a different position of the pipette tip when ejecting sperm in the oocyte is supposed to increase calcium levels during injection and enable better contact of sperm with intracellular storage of calcium.

6. Diagnostic tools for assessing sperm- or oocyte-dependent activation defects

A proper diagnostic procedure is very important prior to the decision to use artificial oocyte activation, and oocyte or sperm donation is a reasonable treatment option for some couples [87].

There are several diagnostic methods available, but not always accessible to all clinics since legislation can prohibit the use of heterologous human-animal models.

The mouse oocyte activation test (MOAT) is a heterologous ICSI model where mouse oocytes are fertilized with the patient's sperm [78]. As a negative control, mouse oocytes are injected with the medium and as a positive control, they are injected with donor sperm with proven fertilizing ability. It allows discrimination between sperm- and oocyte-borne causes for fertilization failure. According to the ratio of fertilized mouse oocytes, three groups are described: MOAT1 indicating sperm-borne defects, MOAT2 fertilization failure of unknown origin, MOAT3 sperm defects are excluded indicating oocyte defects.

In some patients from groups MOAT2 or MOAT3, capacity to activate mouse oocytes is demonstrated but later ICSI-AOA results in TFF. In these cases, assessment of calcium oscillations can give better answers as to whether the underlying reason is the presence of human sperm activation deficiencies or oocyte-related activation deficiency. Mouse oocyte Ca^{2+} analysis (M-OCA) or even more sensitive human oocyte Ca^{2+} analysis (H-OCA) can be performed before using AOA [88]. In the M-OCA test, the patient's sperm is used and frequency patterns of calcium oscillations are analyzed. H-OCA yields higher sensitivity than M-OCA to detect the presence of human sperm activation deficiencies. It helps detect cases with suspected oocyte-related activation deficiency.

7. Success rates of AOA

The systematic review and meta-analysis of RCTs that compared ICSI-AOA and conventional ICSI first established that there is insufficient evidence available from RCTs to judge the efficacy and safety of ICSI-AOA for couples with previous fertilization failure [89]. A total of 14 articles were assessed and 9 included in meta-analysis. It cannot be concluded that the outcomes are improved using ICSI followed by artificial oocyte activation compared with conventional ICSI. The fertilization rate, cleavage rate, and likelihood of blastocyst formation seem to improve according to some studies, but it is difficult to make a general conclusion.

Recently, important evidence appeared that the conditions in which activation takes place are very important for the success rate and can vary a lot. Varying concentrations of both ionomycin and calcium ions in culture media used during AOA can have significant effects on calcium release and further embryonic developmental potential .

8. Safety of AOA methods

Although AOA methods have been proven efficient to overcome some cases of TFF, the concern around using them in clinical practice is quite big. By artificially increasing intracellular calcium levels we interfere with cellular mechanisms that normally would not occur. Nature has regulatory mechanisms to eliminate errors and when we force events that would not happen spontaneously it is always important to verify all possible negative effects of such procedures.

The number of children born after AOA is relatively small for statistical analysis, but there are accumulating data on the safety of these methods. The study from Ghent analyzed neonatal and neurodevelopmental outcomes of 21 children born after cycles with AOA [90]. For all tests and questionnaires, the mean outcomes lay within the expected ranges, but since the number of studied cases is small, the authors state that AOA should still be performed only in selected couples. In another study, 79 children born following AOA-ICSI and 89 born by ICSI were compared in terms of intrauterine fetal death, preterm delivery, birth weight, growth rate, hospitalization in neonatal intensive care units, abnormal behavior according to age, and the physical and mental health of children born and no significant differences were found [91].

In a study, genetic content of donated oocytes in metaphase II artificially activated with calcium-ionophore was analyzed. By using array comparative genomic hybridization, single-nucleotide polymorphism genotyping and maternal haplotyping chromosome segregation errors in meiosis II were not increased compared to the control group [92].

There are concerns about the effects of AOA on gene expression and later embryonic development coming from animal studies [33, 93]. In the case of the use of $SrCl_2$ for AOA, data in mice show that birth weight of male pups is reduced [80].

9. Conclusions

The problem of failed fertilization is a big burden for patients and clinicians and the pressure to help these patients is enormous. Today, ART methods are generally easily accessible and patients' expectations are very high. In Europe alone, there have been 1,308,289 children born from IVF treatments between the years 1997 and 2013 according to data collected in European IVF monitoring [94]. Global data collection on IVF is a difficult task, but there are reports that in a three-year period, more than a million babies are born worldwide [95]. Despite the great success of ART, there are always some patients facing fertilization failure and the emotional burden of inability to achieve pregnancy is great for these couples. For successful fertilization, sperm must activate a quiescent oocyte to complete meiosis and progress toward embryonic development characterized with repeated mitotic divisions. Oocyte activation is a complex cascade of intracellular processes. Sperm or oocyte abnormalities can contribute to activation failure. In clinical practice, there is a need for safe methods of artificial oocyte activation based on the physiological properties of the gametes that closely imitate calcium oscillations triggered naturally by sperm.

Conflict of interest

The authors confirm that there are no known "conflicts of interest" associated with this publication.

Notes/thanks/other declarations

The publication is a part of research program P3-0327 and research project J3-7177 funded by the Slovenian Research Agency.

Author details

Nina Hojnik* and Borut Kovačič
Department of Reproductive Medicine and Gynecological Endocrinology,
University Medical Centre Maribor, Maribor, Slovenia

*Address all correspondence to: hojnina@ukc-mb.si

References

[1] Steptoe PC, Edwards RG. Birth after the reimplantation of a human embryo. Lancet. 1978;**2**(8085):366

[2] Palermo G, Joris H, Devroey P, Van Steirteghem AC. Pregnancies after intracytoplasmic injection of single spermatozoon into an oocyte. Lancet. 1992;**340**(8810):17-18

[3] Sousa M, Tesarik J. Ultrastructural analysis of fertilization failure after intracytoplasmic sperm injection. Human Reproduction. 1994;**9**(12):2374-2380

[4] Flaherty SP, Payne D, Swann NJ, Matthews CD. Aetiology of failed and abnormal fertilization after intracytoplasmic sperm injection. Human Reproduction. 1995;**10**(10):2623-2629

[5] Bhattacharya S, Hamilton MPR, Shaaban M, Khalaf Y, Seddler M, Ghobara T, et al. Conventional in-vitro fertilisation versus intracytoplasmic sperm injection for the treatment of non-male-factor infertility: A randomised controlled trial. Lancet. 2001;**357**(9274):2075-2079

[6] Esfandiari N, Javed MH, Gotlieb L, Casper RF. Complete failed fertilization after intracytoplasmic sperm injection--analysis of 10 years' data. International Journal of Fertility and Women's Medicine. 2005;**50**(4):187-192

[7] Flaherty SP, Payne D, Matthews CD. Fertilization failures and abnormal fertilization after intracytoplasmic sperm injection. Human Reproduction. 1998;**13**(suppl. 1):155-164

[8] Liu J, Nagy Z, Joris H, Tournaye H, Smitz J, Camus M, et al. Analysis of 76 total fertilization failure cycles out of 2732 intracytoplasmic sperm injection cycles. Human Reproduction. 1995;**10**(10):2630-2636

[9] Yanagida K, Morozumi K, Katayose H, Hayashi S, Sato A. Successful pregnancy after ICSI with strontium oocyte activation in low rates of fertilization. Reproductive Biomedicine Online. 2006;**13**(6):801-806

[10] Shinar S, Almog B, Levin I, Shwartz T, Amit A, Hasson J. Total fertilization failure in intra-cytoplasmic sperm injection cycles-classification and management. Gynecological Endocrinology. 2014;**30**(8):593-596

[11] Vlaisavljević V, Kovacic B, Reljic M, Lovrec VG, Sajko MC. Results of intracytoplasmic sperm injection of single oocyte in 362 unstimulated cycles. Journal of Assisted Reproduction and Genetics. 2002;**19**(3):127-131

[12] Dozortsev D, Sutter PD, Dhont M. Fertilization and early embryology: Behaviour of spermatozoa in human oocytes displaying no or one pronucleus after intracytoplasmic sperm injection. Human Reproduction. 1994;**9**(11):2139-2144

[13] Yanagida K. Complete fertilization failure in ICSI. Human Cell. 2004;**17**(4):187-193

[14] Pitsos MA, Nicolopoulou-Stamati P. DNA spatial distribution in unfertilized human oocytes by confocal laser scanning microscope. Molecular Reproduction and Development. 2002;**62**(3):368-374

[15] Kovacic B, Vlaisavljevic V. Configuration of maternal and paternal chromatin and pertaining microtubules in human oocytes failing to fertilize after intracytoplasmic sperm injection. Molecular Reproduction and Development. 2000;**55**(2):197-204

[16] Rawe VY, Olmedo SB, Nodar FN, Doncel GD, Acosta AA, Vitullo AD. Cytoskeletal organization defects

and abortive activation in human oocytes after IVF and ICSI failure. Molecular Human Reproduction. 2000;**6**(6):510-516

[17] Gasca S, Reyftmann L, Pellestor F, Rème T, Assou S, Anahory T, et al. Case report: Total fertilization failure and molecular abnormalities in metaphase II oocytes. Reproductive Biomedicine Online. 2008;**17**(6):772-781

[18] Mazia D. The release of calcium in Arbacia eggs on fertilization. Journal of Cellular and Comparative Physiology. 1937;**10**:291-304

[19] Ridgway EB, Gilkey JC, Jaffe LF. Free calcium increases explosively in activating medaka eggs. Proceedings of the National Academy of Sciences of the United States of America. 1977;**74**(2):623-627

[20] Stricker SA. Comparative biology of calcium signaling during fertilization and egg activation in animals. Developmental Biology. 1999;**211**(2):157-176

[21] Kaneuchi T, Sartain CV, Takeo S, Horner VL, Buehner NA, Aigaki T, et al. Calcium waves occur as *Drosophila* oocytes activate. Proceedings of the National Academy of Sciences. 2015;**112**(3):791-796

[22] Epel D. Mechanisms of activation of sperm and egg during fertilization of sea urchin gametes. Current Topics in Developmental Biology. 1978;**12**(C):185-246

[23] Swann K, Lai FA. Egg activation at fertilization by a soluble sperm protein. Physiological Reviews. 2016;**96**(1):127-149

[24] Miyazaki S. Fertilization potential and calcium transients in mammalian eggs. Development, Growth & Differentiation. 1988;**30**(6):603-610

[25] Igusa Y, Miyazaki S. Effects of altered extracellular and intracellular calcium concentration on hyperpolarizing responses of hamster egg. Journal of Physiology. 1983;**340**:611-632

[26] Taylor CT, Lawrence YM, Kingsland CR, Biljan MM, Cuthbertson KSR. Fertilization and early embryology: Oscillations in intracellular free calcium induced by spermatozoa in human oocytes at fertilization. Human Reproduction. 1993;**8**(12):2174-2179

[27] Gianaroli L, Tosti E, Magli C, Iaccarino M, Ferraretti AP, Dale B. Fertilization current in the human oocyte. Molecular Reproduction and Development. 1994;**38**(2):209-214

[28] Tosti E, Boni R, Cuomo A. Fertilization and activation currents in bovine oocytes. Reproduction. 2002;**124**(6):835-846

[29] Tesarik J, Sousa M, Testart J. Human oocyte activation after intracytoplasmic sperm injection. Human Reproduction. 1994;**9**(3):511-518

[30] Yeste M, Jones C, Amdani SN, Patel S, Coward K. Oocyte activation deficiency: A role for an oocyte contribution? Human Reproduction Update. 2016;**22**(1):23-47

[31] Bos-Mikich A, Whittingham DG, Jones KT. Meiotic and mitotic Ca^{2+} oscillations affect cell composition in resulting blastocysts. Developmental Biology. 1997;**182**(1):172-179

[32] Jones KT. Mammalian egg activation: From Ca^{2+} spiking to cell cycle progression. Reproduction. 2005;**130**(6):813-823

[33] Ducibella T, Schultz RM, Ozil JP. Role of calcium signals in early development. Seminars in Cell & Developmental Biology. 2006;**17**(2):324-332

[34] Kline D. Calcium-dependent events at fertilization of the frog egg: Injection of a calcium buffer blocks ion channel opening, exocytosis, and formation of pronuclei. Developmental Biology. 1988;**126**(2):346-361

[35] Fukuda Y. The time of cortical granule breakdown and sperm penetration in mouse and hamster eggs inseminated in vitro. Biology of Reproduction. 1978;**19**:261-266

[36] Sone Y, Ito M, Shirakawa H, Shikano T, Takeuchi H, Kinoshita K, et al. Nuclear translocation of phospholipase C-zeta, an egg-activating factor, during early embryonic development. Biochemical and Biophysical Research Communications. 2005;**330**(3):690-694

[37] Ducibella T, Huneau D, Angelichio E, Xu Z, Schultz RM, Kopf GS, et al. Egg-to-embryo transition is driven by differential responses to Ca^{2+} oscillation number. Developmental Biology. 2002;**250**(2):280-291

[38] Oliveira AG, Guimaraes ES, Andrade LM, Menezes GB, Fatima LM. Decoding calcium signaling across the nucleus. Physiology. 2014;**29**(5):361-368

[39] Santella L, Lim D, Moccia F. Calcium and fertilization: The beginning of life. Trends in Biochemical Sciences. 2004;**29**(8):400-408

[40] Dale B. Is the idea of a fast block to polyspermy based on artifact? Biochemical and Biophysical Research Communications. 2014;**450**(3):1159-1165

[41] Dale B, Wilding M, Coppola G, Tosti E. How do spermatozoa activate oocytes? Reproductive Biomedicine Online. 2010;**21**(1):1-3

[42] Tosti E, Boni R. Electrical events during gamete maturation and fertilization in animals and humans. Human Reproduction Update. 2004;**10**(1):53-65

[43] Brezina PR, Yunus FN, Zhao Y. Effects of pharmaceutical medications on male fertility. Journal of Reproduction & Infertility. 2012;**13**(1):3-11

[44] Nomikos M, Swann K, Lai FA. Starting a new life: Sperm PLC-zeta mobilizes the Ca^{2+} signal that induces egg activation and embryo development: An essential phospholipase C with implications for male infertility. BioEssays. 2012;**34**(2):126-134

[45] Swann K. A cytosolic sperm factor stimulates repetitive calcium increases and mimics fertilization in hamster eggs. Development. 1990;**110**(4):1295-1302

[46] Stricker SA. Intracellular injections of a soluble sperm factor trigger calcium oscillations and meiotic maturation in unfertilized oocytes of a marine worm. Developmental Biology. 1997;**186**(2):185-201

[47] Parrington J, Swann K, Shevchenko VI, Sesay AK, Lai FA. Calcium oscillations in mammalian eggs triggered by a soluble sperm protein. Nature. 1996;**379**:364

[48] Carroll DJ, Albay DT, Terasaki M, Jaffe LA, Foltz KR. Identification of PLC y-dependent and -independent events during fertilization of eggs. Developmental Biology. 1999;**206**(2):232-247

[49] Kuo RC, Baxter GT, Thompson SH, Stricker SA, Patton C, Bonaventura J, et al. NO is necessary and sufficient for egg activation at fertilization. Nature. 2000;**406**(6796):633-636

[50] Wu ATH, Sutovsky P, Manandhar G, Xu W, Katayama M, Day BN, et al. PAWP, a sperm-specific WW

domain-binding protein, promotes meiotic resumption and pronuclear development during fertilization. The Journal of Biological Chemistry. 2007;**282**(16):12164-12175

[51] Rice A, Parrington J, Jones KT, Swann K. Mammalian sperm contain a Ca^{2+}–sensitive phospholipase C activity that can generate InsP3from PIP2associated with intracellular organelles. Developmental Biology. 2000;**228**(1):125-135

[52] Saunders CM, Larman MG, Parrington J, Cox LJ, Royse J, Blayney LM, et al. PLC zeta: A sperm-specific trigger of Ca(2+) oscillations in eggs and embryo development. Development. 2002;**129**(15):3533-3544

[53] Escoffier J, Yassine S, Lee HC, Martinez G, Delaroche J, Coutton C, et al. Subcellular localization of phospholipase Cζ in human sperm and its absence in DPY19L2-deficient sperm are consistent with its role in oocyte activation. MHR: Basic Science of Reproductive Medicine. 2015;**21**(2):157-168

[54] Knott JG, Kurokawa M, Fissore RA, Schultz RM, Williams CJ. Transgenic RNA interference reveals role for mouse sperm phospholipase Cζ in triggering Ca^{2+} oscillations during Fertilization1. Biology of Reproduction. 2005;**72**(4):992-996

[55] Escoffier J, Lee HC, Yassine S, Zouari R, Martinez G, Karaouzène T, et al. Homozygous mutation of PLCZ1 leads to defective human oocyte activation and infertility that is not rescued by the WW-binding protein PAWP. Human Molecular Genetics. 2016;**25**(5):878-891

[56] Kashir J, Heindryckx B, Jones C, de Sutter P, Parrington J, Coward K. Oocyte activation, phospholipase C zeta and human infertility. Human Reproduction Update. 2010;**16**(6):690-703

[57] Kashir J, Deguchi R, Jones C, Coward K, Stricker SA. Comparative biology of sperm factors and fertilization-induced calcium signals across the animal kingdom. Molecular Reproduction and Development. 2013;**80**(10):787-815

[58] Faure JE, Myles DG, Primakoff P. The frequency of calcium oscillations in mouse eggs at fertilization is modulated by the number of fused sperm. Developmental Biology. 1999;**213**(2):370-377

[59] Hachem A, Godwin J, Ruas M, Lee HC, Ferrer Buitrago M, Ardestani G, et al. PLCζ is the physiological trigger of the Ca^{2+} oscillations that induce embryogenesis in mammals but conception can occur in its absence. Development. 2017;**144**(16):2914-2924

[60] Nasr-Esfahani MH, Razavi S, Mardani M, Shirazi R, Javanmardi S. Effects of failed oocyte activation and sperm protamine deficiency on fertilization post-ICSI. Reproductive Biomedicine Online. 2007;**14**(4):422-429

[61] Nasr-Esfahani MH, Naghshizadian N, Imani H, Razavi S, Mardani M, Kazemi S, et al. Can sperm protamine deficiency induce sperm premature chromosomal condensation? Andrologia. 2006;**38**(3):92-98

[62] Motta PM, Nottola SA, Micara G, Familiari G. Ultrastructure of human unfertilized oocytes and Polyspermic embryos in an IVF-ET program. Annals of the New York Academy of Sciences. 1988;**541**(1):367-383

[63] Liu M. The biology and dynamics of mammalian cortical granules. Reproductive Biology and Endocrinology. 2011;**9**(1):149

[64] Hsieh RH, Tsai NM, Au HK, Chang SJ, Wei YH, Tzeng CR. Multiple rearrangements of mitochondrial DNA

in unfertilized human oocytes. Fertility and Sterility. 2002;**77**(5):1012-1017

[65] FitzHarris G, Marangos P, Carroll J. Changes in endoplasmic reticulum structure during mouse oocyte maturation are controlled by the cytoskeleton and cytoplasmic dynein. Developmental Biology. 2007;**305**(1):133-144

[66] Wakai T, Vanderheyden V, Yoon S-Y, Cheon B, Zhang A, Parys JB, et al. Regulation of inositol 1,4,5-trisphosphate receptor function during mouse oocyte maturation. Journal of Cellular Physiology. 2012;**227**(2):705-717

[67] Ajduk A, Małagocki A, Maleszewski M. Cytoplasmic maturation of mammalian oocytes: Development of a mechanism responsible for sperm-induced Ca^{2+} oscillations. Reproductive Biology. 2008;**8**(1):3-22

[68] Archacka K, Ajduk A, Pomorsiki P, Szczepanska K, Maleszewski M, Ciemerych MA. Defective calcium release during in vitro fertilization of maturing oocytes of LT/Sv mice. International Journal of Developmental Biology. 2008;**52**(7):903-912

[69] Calafell JM, Badenas J, Egozcue J, Santaló J. Premature chromosome condensation as a sign of oocyte immaturity. Human Reproduction. 1991;**6**(7):1017-1021

[70] Sedó CA, Miguens M, Andreucci S, Ortiz N, Lorenzi D, Papier S, et al. Correlation between cytoplamic oocyte maturation and chromosomal aneuploidies—Impact on fertilization, embryo quality and pregnancy. JBRA Assisted Reproduction. 2015;**19**(2):59-65

[71] Lu Y, Ferrer-Buitrago M, Popovic M, Neupane J, De Vos WH, Lierman S, et al. Patients with a high proportion of immature and meiotically resistant oocytes experience defective nuclear oocyte maturation patterns and impaired pregnancy outcomes. Reproductive Biomedicine Online. 2018;**36**(4):396-407

[72] Grindler NM, Moley KH. Maternal obesity, infertility and mitochondrial dysfunction: Potential mechanisms emerging from mouse model systems. Molecular Human Reproduction. 2013;**19**(8):486-494

[73] Mansour R, Fahmy I, Tawab NA, Kamal A, El-Demery Y, Aboulghar M, et al. Electrical activation of oocytes after intracytoplasmic sperm injection: A controlled randomized study. Fertility and Sterility. 2009;**91**(1):133-139

[74] Egashira A, Murakami M, Haigo K, Horiuchi T, Kuramoto T. A successful pregnancy and live birth after intracytoplasmic sperm injection with globozoospermic sperm and electrical oocyte activation. Fertility and Sterility. 2009;**92**(6):2037.e5-2037.e9

[75] Tanaka A, Nagayoshi M, Takemoto Y, Tanaka I, Kusunoki H, Watanabe S, et al. Fourteen babies born after round spermatid injection into human oocytes. Proceedings of the National Academy of Sciences. 2015;**112**(47):14629-14634

[76] Nikiforaki D, Vanden Meerschaut F, De Roo C, Lu Y, Ferrer-Buitrago M, De Sutter P, et al. Effect of two assisted oocyte activation protocols used to overcome fertilization failure on the activation potential and calcium releasing pattern. Fertility and Sterility. 2016;**105**(3):798-806e2

[77] Tesarik J, Nagy ZP, Mendoza C, Greco E. Chemically and mechanically induced membrane fusion: Non-activating methods for nuclear transfer in mature human oocytes. Human Reproduction. 2000;**15**(5):1149-1154

[78] Heindryckx B, Van der Elst J, De Sutter P, Dhont M. Treatment option for

sperm- or oocyte-related fertilization failure: Assisted oocyte activation following diagnostic heterologous ICSI. Human Reproduction. 2005;**20**(8):2237-2241

[79] Nakagawa K, Yamano S, Moride N, Yamashita M, Yoshizawa M, Aono T. Effect of activation with Ca ionophore A23187 and puromycin on the development of human oocytes that failed to fertilize after intracytoplasmic sperm injection. Fertility and Sterility. 2001;**76**(1):148-152

[80] Vanden Meerschaut F, Nikiforaki D, De Roo C, Lierman S, Qian C, Schmitt-John T, et al. Comparison of pre-and post-implantation development following the application of three artificial activating stimuli in a mouse model with round-headed sperm cells deficient for oocyte activation. Human Reproduction. 2013;**28**(5):1190-1198

[81] Kim J-W, Kim S-D, Yang S-H, Yoon S-H, Jung J-H, Lim J-H. Successful pregnancy after SrCl2 oocyte activation in couples with repeated low fertilization rates following calcium ionophore treatment. Systems Biology in Reproductive Medicine. 2014;**60**(3):177-182

[82] Kashir J, Jones C, Lee HC, Rietdorf K, Nikiforaki D, Durrans C, et al. Loss of activity mutations in phospholipase C zeta (PLCzeta) abolishes calcium oscillatory ability of human recombinant protein in mouse oocytes. Human Reproduction. 2011;**26**(12):3372-3387

[83] Yoon S-Y, Eum JH, Lee JE, Lee HC, Kim YS, Han JE, et al. Recombinant human phospholipase C zeta 1 induces intracellular calcium oscillations and oocyte activation in mouse and human oocytes. Human Reproduction. 2012;**27**(6):1768-1780

[84] Grabiec A, Max A, Tischner M. Parthenogenetic activation of domestic cat oocytes using ethanol, calcium ionophore, cycloheximide and a magnetic field. Theriogenology. 2007;**67**(4):795-800

[85] Ebner T, Moser M, Sommergruber M, Jesacher K, Tews G. Complete oocyte activation failure after ICSI can be overcome by a modified injection technique. Human Reproduction. 2004;**19**(8):1837-1841

[86] Tesarik J, Rienzi L, Ubaldi F, Mendoza C, Greco E. Use of a modified intracytoplasmic sperm injection technique to overcome sperm-borne and oocyte-borne oocyte activation failures. Fertility and Sterility. 2002;**78**(3):619-624

[87] Combelles CMH, Morozumi K, Yanagimachi R, Zhu L, Fox JH, Racowsky C. Diagnosing cellular defects in an unexplained case of total fertilization failure. Human Reproduction. 2010;**25**(7):1666-1671

[88] Ferrer-Buitrago M, Dhaenens L, Lu Y, Bonte D, Vanden Meerschaut F, De Sutter P, et al. Human oocyte calcium analysis predicts the response to assisted oocyte activation in patients experiencing fertilization failure after ICSI. Human Reproduction. 2018;**33**(3):416-425

[89] Sfontouris IA, Nastri CO, Lima MLS, Tahmasbpourmarzouni E, Raine-Fenning N, Martins WP. Artificial oocyte activation to improve reproductive outcomes in women with previous fertilization failure: A systematic review and meta-analysis of RCTs. Human Reproduction. 2015;**30**(8):1831-1841

[90] Vanden Meerschaut F, D'Haeseleer E, Gysels H, Thienpont Y, Dewitte G, Heindryckx B, et al. Neonatal and neurodevelopmental outcome of children aged 3-10 years born following assisted oocyte activation. Reproductive Biomedicine Online. 2014;**28**(1):54-63

[91] Deemeh MR, Tavalaee M, Nasr-Esfahani MH. Health of children born through artificial oocyte activation: A pilot study. Reproductive Sciences. 2015;**22**(3):322-328

[92] Capalbo A, Ottolini CS, Griffin DK, Ubaldi FM, Handyside AH, Rienzi L. Artificial oocyte activation with calcium ionophore does not cause a widespread increase in chromosome segregation errors in the second meiotic division of the oocyte. Fertility and Sterility. 2016;**105**(3):807-814e2

[93] Ozil J-P, Banrezes B, Toth S, Pan H, Schultz RM. Ca^{2+} oscillatory pattern in fertilized mouse eggs affects gene expression and development to term. Developmental Biology. 2006;**300**(2):534-544

[94] Calhaz-Jorge C, De Geyter C, Kupka MS, De Mouzon J, Erb K, Mocanu E, et al. Assisted reproductive technology in Europe, 2013: Results generated from European registers by ESHRE. Human Reproduction. 2017;**32**(10):1957-1973

[95] Dyer S, Chambers GM, De Mouzon J, Nygren KG, Zegers-Hochschild F, Mansour R, et al. International committee for monitoring assisted reproductive technologies world report: Assisted reproductive technology 2008, 2009 and 2010. Human Reproduction. 2016;**31**(7):1588-1609

Section 3

Embryo Development and Implantation

Chapter 5

Human Blastocyst Formation and Development

Hilma Putri Lubis and Binarwan Halim

Abstract

The preimplantation period of human embryo development is remarkable and characterized by successive changes in terms of genetic control, physiology, and morphology of the embryo. Human preimplantation embryo development is characterized by the initial phase of embryo development, the phase before the embryo implantation process. In normal conditions, after fertilization, the embryo grows until the blastocyst stage. The blastocyst grows as the cells divide and the cavity expands, where it "hatches" from the zona pellucida to implant into the endometrium. Reprogramming and programming are continuous processes in the embryo that encompasses fusion of the egg and sperm pronuclei; epigenetic reprogramming and modification, an extensive wave of degradation of maternal transcripts, and activation of the nascent human embryonic genome and aneuploidy can occur in this stage. The embryo produces cytokines, growth factors, and receptors for endometrial signals in the apposition stage.

Keywords: preimplantation, embryo, epigenetic, reprogramming, blastocyst

1. Introduction

Preimplantation embryo development is characterized by a series of events after fertilization including the formation of the maternal and paternal pronuclei, followed by the formation of the zygote, which at ±20 hours after insemination starts undergoing mitotic divisions every 12–18 hours (cleavage stage), reaching the morula (compaction), and the blastocyst grows as the cells divide and the cavity expands, until it arrives at the uterus, where it "hatches" from the zona pellucida to implant into the endometrium. The main objective of blastocyst culture was to increase the success rate of in vitro fertilization (IVF) because of better embryo selection. Blastocyst culture has also been used as a tool to select the most viable embryos in a cohort with a consequent reduction in the number of embryos transferred and the corresponding reduction in the incidence of multiple gestations. This chapter will review about human blastocyst formation and development and discuss about the physiology, morphology, and gene expression of the blastocyst.

2. Physiology of the blastocyst

The transformation of the fertilized oocyte into the blastocyst is not only characterized by major morphological events but also by dramatic changes in its

IntechOpen

physiology, reflected in changes in the relative activity of the metabolic pathways which provide not only energy but also the biosynthetic intermediates required to support proliferation [1]. The ability of the cleavage stage embryo to react in the environment during early cleavage is limited because the human genome embryo is still inactive and the system that regulates the balance of the osmotic pressure is not fully functional [1, 2].

The tendency of metabolism to produce energy from pronucleate oocytes until blastocyst stage can be assessed from mitochondrial forms. In the stage of pronucleate oocytes and cleavage stage, their mitochondrial form is still immature, and the production of energy in oocytes is usually low and will be increased tremendously from cleavage stage embryo until blastocyst stage. In the stage of pronucleate oocytes, the type of metabolism is oxidative phosphorylation (OXPHOST); then in the cleavage stage embryo, the metabolism uses lactate, pyruvate, specific amino acids, and fatty acids [1–3].

In the blastocyst stage, the metabolism produces energy that mainly depends on the process of glycolysis, with anabolic dominantly seen in the mitochondria [3, 4].

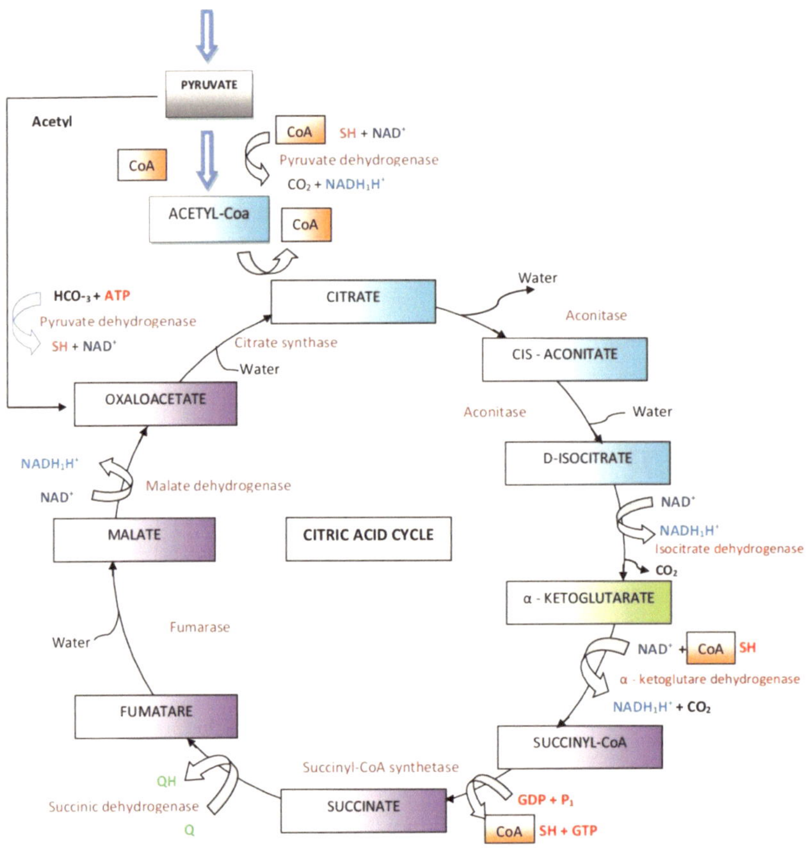

Figure 1.

Tricarboxylic acid (TCA) cycle or the Krebs cycle. The citric acid cycle begins with one acetyl-CoA molecule reacting with one molecule of H2O, releasing a coenzyme-A group, and donating the remaining two carbon atoms in the form of an acetyl group to oxaloacetic acid which has molecules with four carbon atoms, to produce citric acid with six carbon atoms. The outcome products of the first turn of the cycle are one GTP (or ATP), three NADH, one QH_2, and two CO_2. Because two acetyl-CoA molecules are produced from each glucose molecule, two cycles are required per glucose molecule. Therefore, at the end of two cycles, the final products are two GTP, six NADH, two QH_2, and four CO_2.

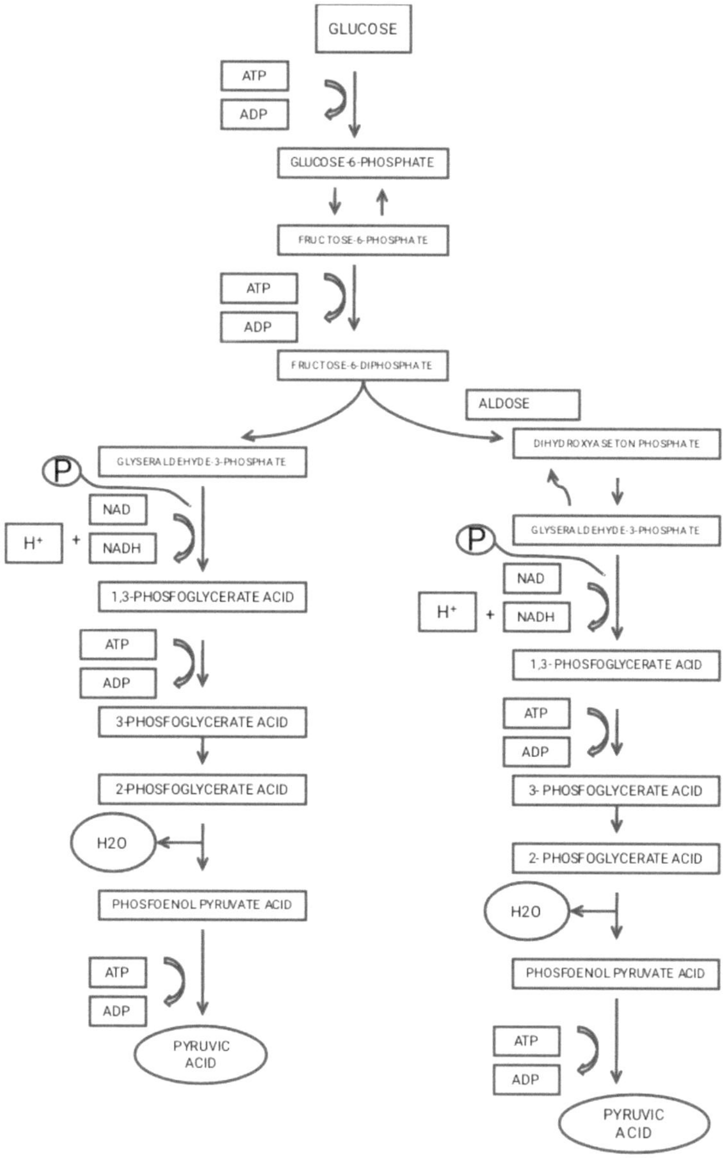

Figure 2.

Glycolysis pathway or Embden-Meyerhof-Parnas (EMP) pathway. (1) In the first stage, glucose will be converted to glucose 6-phosphate by the hexokinase enzyme. This stage requires energy from adenosine triphosphate (ATP). The ATP that has released the stored energy will change to ADP. (2) Glucose 6-phosphate will be converted to fructose 6-phosphate which is catalyzed by the enzyme phosphohexose isomerase. (3) Fructose 6-phosphate will be converted to fructose 1,6-bisphosphate; this reaction is catalyzed by the enzyme phosphofructokinase. In this reaction, energy from ATP is needed. (4) Fructose 1,6-bisphosphate (6 C atoms) will be broken down into glyceraldehyde 3-phosphate (3 atoms C) and dihydroxy acetone phosphate (3 atoms C). The reaction is catalyzed by the enzyme aldolase. (5) One molecule of dihydroxy acetone phosphate that is formed will be converted to glyceraldehyde 3-phosphate by the enzyme triose phosphate isomerase. The enzyme works back and forth, meaning it can also convert glyceraldehyde 3-phosphate to dihydroxy acetone phosphate. (6) Glyceraldehyde 3-phosphate will then be converted to 1,3-bisphosphoglycerate by the enzyme glyceraldehyde 3-phosphate dehydrogenase. In this reaction NADH will be formed. (7) 1,3 bisphosphoglycerate will be converted to 3-phosphoglycerate by the phosphoglycerate kinase enzyme. These reactions will be released as energy in the form of ATP. (8) 3-phosphoglycerate will be converted into 2-phosphoglycerate by the phosphoglycerate mutase enzyme. (9) 2-phosphoglycerate will be converted to phosphoenolpyruvate by the enzyme enolase. (10) Phosphoenolpyruvate will be converted to pyruvate which is catalyzed by the pyruvate kinase enzyme. In this stage also produced energy in the form of ATP.

In the cleavage stage embryo, pyruvate uptake increases continuously until the blastocyst stage. In the blastocyst stage, glucose uptake is higher than pyruvate uptake, and O_2 consumption will increase in the initial development stage before compaction (pre-compaction). In the pre-compaction stage, we can observe low biosynthetic activity, low O_2 consumption, and ovoid form of mitochondria; the main nutrition is pyruvate, with dominant maternal genome where cells divide in the similar shape [1–3].

In the post-compaction stage, we can observe high biosynthetic activity, higher oxygen consumption, and elongated form of mitochondria; the main nutrition is glucose, and with dominant human embryo genome. In this stage, cells will be differentiated into trophectoderm (TE) and inner cell mass (ICM) [1–3, 5].

Amino acids in the metabolism of blastocyst can be used as a source of energy, and some amino acids such as aspartate through malate aspartate shuttle enter in the tricarboxylic acid (TCA) cycle to produce energy. However, glutamine can also

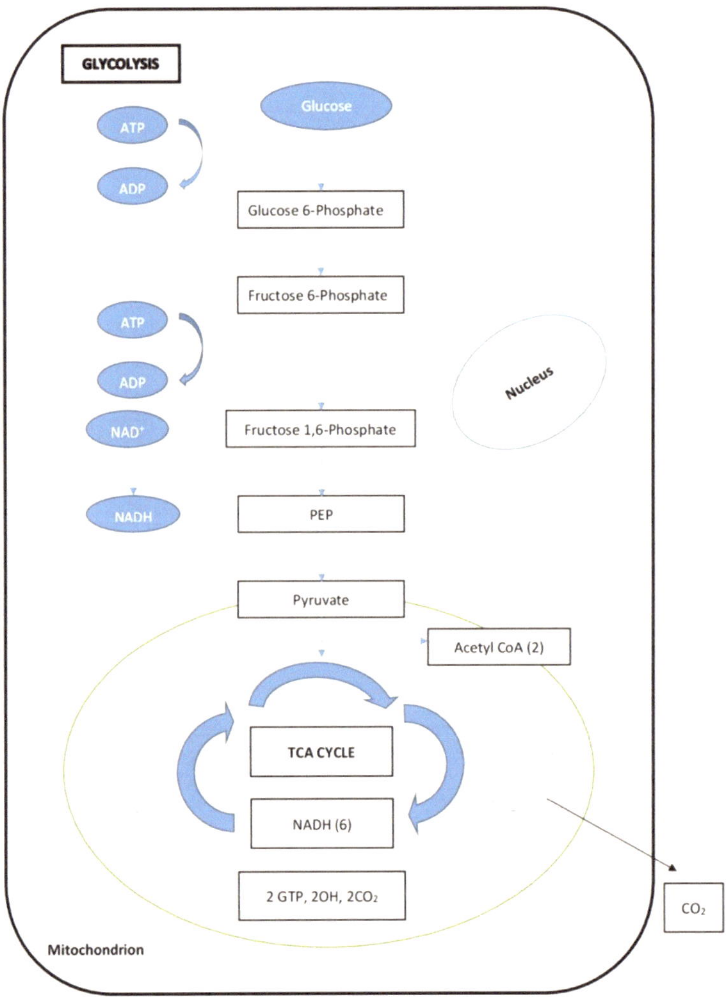

Figure 3.
Metabolism of the blastocyst. After compaction, there is an increase in oxygen consumption and utilization of glucose as a source of energy (glycolysis). The increase in oxygen consumption reflects the considerable energy required for the formation and maintenance of the blastocoel, but the increase in glucose utilization reflects an increased demand for biosynthetic process. In TCA cycles, it produces NADH, GTP, QH, and CO_2 and 34 ATP. PEP, phosphoenolpyruvate.

enter as glutamate in the TCA cycle to produce energy. Amino acid in the blastocyst stage also plays a role in the regulation of intracellular pH buffer, as a material development process and as antioxidants and chelators [1–3, 5].

After compaction, the embryo exhibits increased of O_2 consumption and glucose usage capacity as an energy source. This oxygen consumption increase shows that the energy is needed for the formation and maintenance of blastocoel [1–3, 5].

Increased metabolism of the blastocyst occurs due to the increased release of blastomere to 150–200 cells with the formation and maintenance of blastocoel through the activity of Na^+/K^+ ATPase pump which produces energy. Energy is needed for the degradation of the zona pellucida with protease enzyme. Pyruvate as a source of energy reserves other than carbohydrates also functions as an antioxidant [1–3, 5].

The human blastocyst uses amino acids as a source of energy in the catabolism process and produces ammonium 30 pmol/hour. The most used amino acid is aspartate, besides consuming arginine, serine, methionine, valine, and leucine [1–3, 5].

Metabolism of the blastocyst occurs in two different places: in trophectoderm (TE) cells where glucose consumption occurs and half is converted to lactate, whereas glycolysis process occurs in inner cell mass (ICM) (**Figures 1–3**) [1–3, 5].

3. Morphology of the blastocyst

In in vitro fertilization (IVF), the blastocyst culture was important to increase the success rate of IVF because of better embryo selection after better genomic activation and endometrial receptivity [6]. The blastocyst comprises two cell types: the inner cell mass (ICM, from which the fetal tissues develop) and the trophectoderm (which will form mostly extraembryonic tissues such as the placenta [1]). This morphological differentiation was thought to represent the developmental capability of the blastocyst [6, 7].

3.1 Degree of expansion

The fluid accumulation presence between cells at the morulae stage is the phase that determines embryonic development. The accumulated fluid will form blastocoel gradually which usually occurs on day 4 and/or on the beginning of day 5 human embryo stage which marks the development of new embryos known as the blastocyst stage. An increase in fluid volume and the number of cells in the blastocyst causes an enhancement in the size cavity of the blastocyst and its cavity with depletion of the zona pellucida (ZP) [6]. The number of cells that comprise a blastocyst can vary considerably as shown in one study to range between 24 and 322 cells, which is often reflected in the blastocyst's morphology [8].

The stages of blastocyst embryo development are divided into four grades. A grade of 1 is given to the embryo with blastocoel cavity less than 50% of the embryo volume. A grade of 2 is given to the embryo with blastocoel cavity as much as 50% of the embryo volume or even more than that. A grade of 3 was given to the embryo that had a blastocoel cavity which had fulfilled that all embryos and zona pellucida (ZP) appeared to be thinner than embryo on day 3. A grade of 4 is given to the embryo that has successfully hatched from ZP [6, 9].

3.2 ICM morphology

A collection of cells located within the blastocoel in one pole of the blastocyst cavity is called ICM. ICM will develop into fetal tissue. ICM consists of tightly packed cells and loosely bound cells that cause the size of the ICM very large and/or small morphologically [6]. The morphological form of ICM is assessed based on how much the cell compaction is until there is no cell clot at all. A grade of 1 is given to ICM with a very large and dense form of cell clots. A grade of 2 is given to ICM with a slightly diffuse cell form. A grade of 3 is given to ICM with very few cells and which does not even form clots. However, the best ICM grade (A) contains tightly packed and many cells; the middle ICM grade (B) is composed of loosely grouped and several cells, and the worst grade (C) describes an ICM that contains very few cells that are loosely bound [6, 9].

3.3 TE morphology

The outer cells of the blastocyst, forming the blastocyst structure itself, are called the trophectoderm (TE) cells. TE cells play a role in the formation of fluid accumulation in the blastocoel which can be a key in ICM determination, but in the early stages of the blastocyst stage, the role of TE cells is unclear. TE cells will develop into extraembryonic tissue such as the placenta. In addition, TE cells are thought to play a role in the implantation process which the TE cells have contributed in the phase of apposition, adhesion, and invasion of the endometrium which can support the implantation of the blastocyst in the uterus. Molecular factors are also produced by TE cells that play a role in the embryo implantation process [6–9]. The TE cells have traditionally been graded in a similar manner to the ICM, i.e., by their number and cohesiveness according to three different grades (A, B, C). According to blastocyst grading by Gardner and Schoolcraft, the best TE cell grade (A) contains many cells that form a cohesive epithelium; the middle TE category (B) is composed of few cells forming a loose epithelium, and the worst category (C) describes a TE that contains very few large cells that struggle to form a cohesive epithelium. However, other publications have found no relationship between TE grade and viability (**Figure 4**) [6, 8, 9].

Gardner and Schoolcraft in 1999 introduced the blastocyst grading system which is adopted by the majority of IVF laboratories in the world. In the blastocyst grading system, they classified the degree of blastocyst into three category,

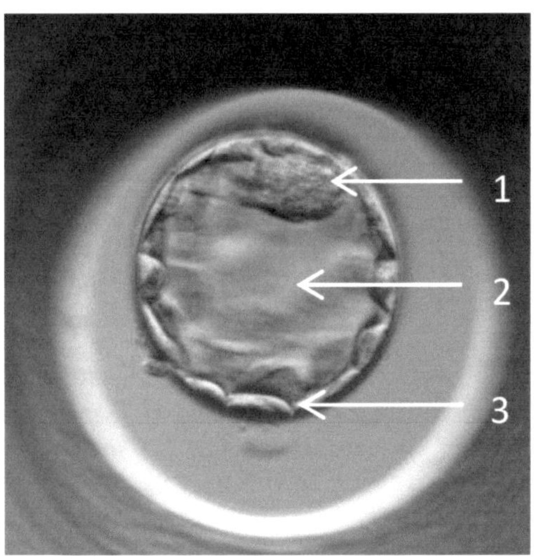

Figure 4.
Blastocyst morphology. (1) inner cell mass (ICM), (2) blastocoel, and (3) trophectoderm.

DOI: http://dx.doi.org/10.5772/intechopen.82095

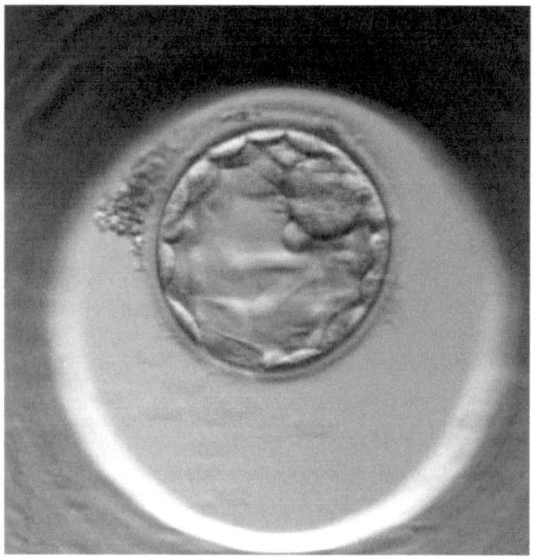

Figure 5.
Blastocyst (grade 4: A: A) means that the blastocyst has been expanded (grade 4), has a large ICM and compact (grade A), and has TE which consists of many cells which are mutually binding (grade A).

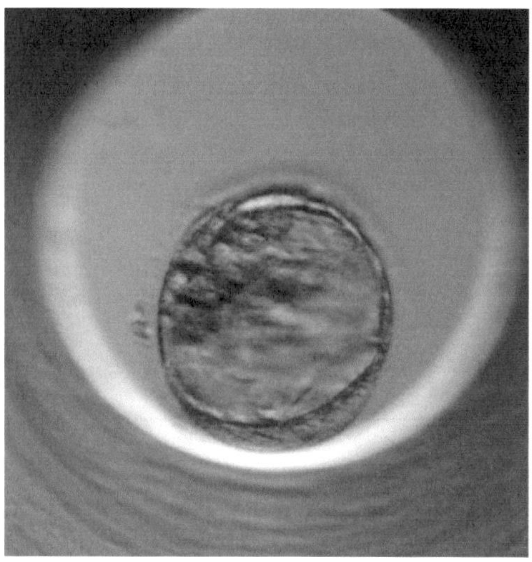

Figure 6.
Blastocyst (grade 4: C: C) means that blastocyst embryo has been expanded (grade 4), has ICM that is difficult to see and has very few cells (grade C), and has TE which has very little cell (grade C).

i.e., degree of expansion, inner cell mass (ICM) quality, and the trophectoderm (TE) cell quality [6, 10].

Alpha Scientists in Reproductive Medicine and ESHRE Special Interest Group of Embryology states that a good embryo on day 5 which is examined at 116 ± 2 hours must be in the form of blastocyst [9].

Embryo, according to the Istanbul consensus, is given a grade based on three things; the first thing is the embryo development stage, the second is ICM, and the third is TE. So that the order of the fifth day embryo assessment is based on the stages of development, then based on ICM morphology, and the last is based on TE. The following is a presentation of the fifth day embryo according to the Istanbul consensus (**Figures 5–9; Table 1**) [6, 9].

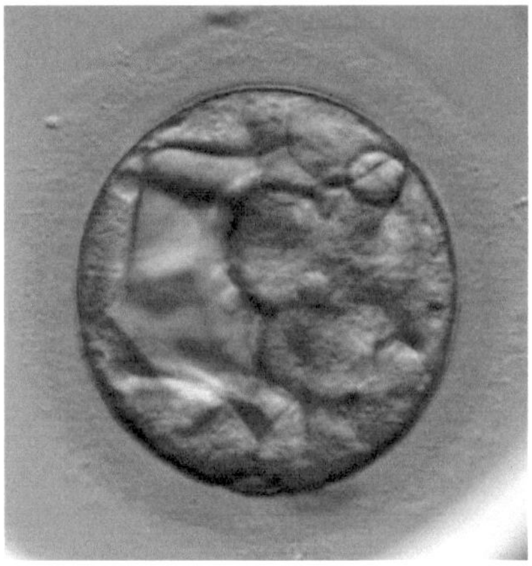

Figure 7.
Early blastocyst is the fifth day embryo development stage which has a blastocoel less than 50% of the embryo volume, and the formation of ICM and TE is not clear.

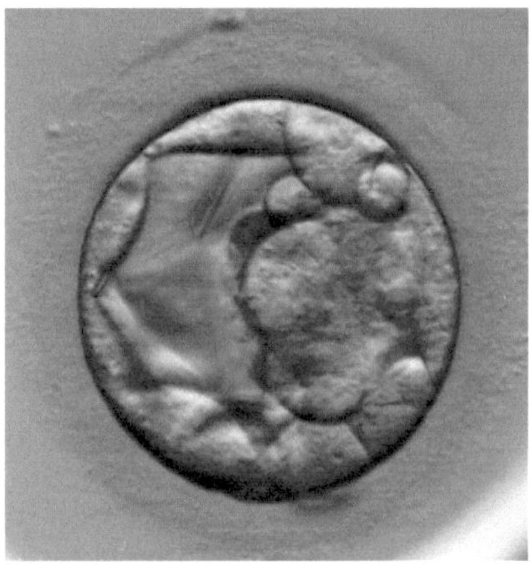

Figure 8.
Blastocyst (grade 2: A: A) embryos that have embryo development stage with a grade of 2 are blastocyst embryos which still have thick ZP.

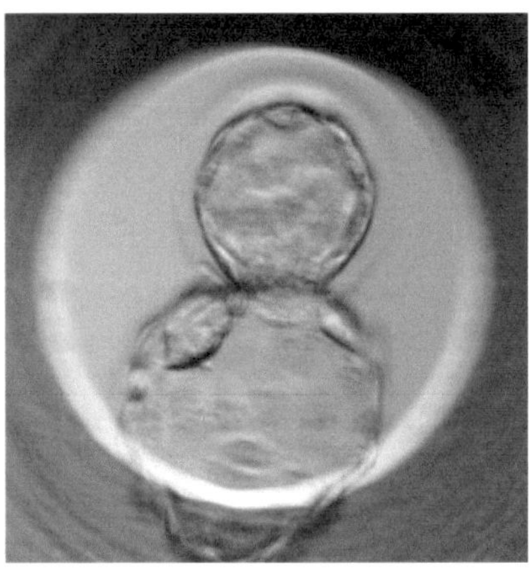

Figure 9.
Blastocyst (grade 5: A: A) means that blastocyst embryo which has come out of its shell (grade 5) has ICM whose cells are large and easy to observe (grade A) and has TE consisting of many cells (grade A).

Expansion grade	**Blastocyst development and stage status**
1	Early blastocyst—Blastocoel cavity less than half the volume of the embryo
2	Blastocyst—Blastocoel cavity more than half the volume of the embryo
3	Full blastocyst—Blastocoel completely filling the embryo
4	Expanded blastocyst—Blastocoel volume is now larger than that of early embryo and zona is thinner
5	Hatching out of the shell
6	Hatched out of the shell
ICM grade	**Inner cell mass quality**
A	Tightly packed and many cells
B	Loosely grouped and several cells
C	Very few cells
TE grade	**Trophectoderm quality**
A	Many cells forming a cohesive epithelium
B	Few cells forming a loose epithelium
C	Very few large cells

Table 1.
The blastocyst grading system. Modified from Gardner and Schoolcraft.

4. Gene expression of human preimplantation embryo

The human embryo preimplantation development is characterized by reprogramming and programming that encompasses fusion of the egg and sperm pronuclei, epigenetic reprogramming, an extensive wave of degradation of maternal transcripts, and activation of the nascent human embryonic genome [11, 12].

There are 1909 genes expressed in only oocytes (maternal genome) and 3122 genes expressed in only blastocyst (embryonic genome). The main difference in observed profile expression between oocytes and embryos is reflected in blastocyst and oocyte specific gene expression analysis. Specific oocyte and blastocyst genes are separated in groups by expression levels. There are 270 specific oocyte genes and 308 blastocyst-specific genes that show high levels of expression. In the panther pathway analysis of high expression genes, the MII oocyte pathway is Wnt signaling pathway, where blastocyst-specific genes are expressed according to integrin signaling pathway, cytoskeletal regulation. The scarcity of the materials, however, both in size (10.1 mm diameter) and in quantity (only a few to tens of oocytes from each ovulation), have been almost the molecular analysis of preimplantation embryos [11–13].

Some interesting patterns in embryo preimplantation based on transcriptional genome-wide analysis include: (1) several genes that experience up- or downregulation during human oocyte maturation from immature germinal vesicle oocyte to the oocyte metaphase II stage; (2) partially expressed transcripts of the MII oocytes will be partially downregulated or degraded during the development to the 4-cell stage; (3) many genes are upregulated after the 4-cell stage, which reflects the main wave Embryonic Genome Activation (EGA); (4) genes involved in lineage commitment are regulated in the development of preimplantation; and (5) many expressed genes dynamically encode transcription factors, epigenetic modifying factors, and chromatin remodeling [12–16].

Human genome activation begins in the 4- and 8-cell stages or even in the early 2-cell stage. Data suggest that TE or ICM cell lineage-associated genes are expressed in human embryos later than in mice at around early blastocyst stage, but it is still unclear. Human embryos can be cultured in vitro for 7–8 days post-fertilization. Genes unique in the blastocysts included annexins A2 and A3 (ANXA2, ANXA3), gap junction protein alpha 1 (GJPA1), guanosine triphosphate-binding protein 4 (GTPBP4), and adenosine triphosphatase H.–transporting, lysosomal accessory protein 1 (ATP6AP1). The blastocyst-specific genes were associated with oxidative phosphorylation, glycolysis, and sterol metabolism and were rich in RNA-binding proteins, methyltransferases, gap junction proteins, and intermediate filaments. Oxidative phosphorylation and glycolysis processes control ATP generation during pre-compaction and cavitation stages, respectively. Highly expressed blastocyst genes were involved in the Rho GTPase, control pathway that regulates cytoskeletal changes occurring during cell growth and development; the PDGF pathway, which plays a critical role in cellular proliferation and metabolism, and the integrin signaling pathway are also important in actin reorganization [12–19].

Studies on gene expression during the preimplantation period have identified transcription factors from housekeeping genes, transcription and growth factor genes, sex-determining genes, tissues specifics, novel genes, and genes of unknown functions [12, 13].

4.1 Housekeeping gene

Housekeeping gene is a gene that plays a role in regulating basal cell function which is important in cell maintenance and also has a specific role in tissues or organisms. Therefore, housekeeping gene is estimated to be expressed in all cells of organism normally, including tissue, external signal, cell cycle, or cell development stage [12, 13, 20].

Beta-actin, keratin-18, ubiquitous cytoskeletal elements, cell adhesion molecules, and alpha tubulin have been detected, as well as such housekeeping genes as hypoxanthine phosphoribosyl transferase (HPRT), adenosine phosphoribosyl transferase (APRT), glucose-6-phosphate dehydrogenase, hexokinase I, and adenosine deaminase. Overall, out of the 536 housekeeping genes investigated, 427 were detected in the oocyte and 452 in the blastocyst [12, 13, 20].

4.2 Transcription and growth factor genes

Transcription regulators, growth factors, proto-oncogenes cycle gene cells, and receptors are several genes that expressed during the preimplantation period, including CD44, a cell surface glycoprotein that can play a role in implantation; OCT 4 and OCT 6, transcriptional regulators; cyclin B1, a cell cycle gene; colony stimulating factor 1 receptor, c-fms; tumor necrosis factor and its receptors; interleukin-1 type I receptor (IL-1R tI); growth factors such as insulin and their receptors; epidermal growth factor receptor (EGF-R), epidermal growth factor (EGF), and transformation of growth factor-alpha (TGF-α) [12, 13, 17–19].

4.3 Tissue-specific genes, novel genes, and genes of unknown function

A major histocompatibility complex molecule was detected in preimplantation human embryos and implicated tissue-specific genes as globin and interleukin-10 and also human transposable element, LINE-1, and known expressed sequence tags

(ESTs) in the GenBank and dbEST databases. Of the 46 peptide hormone genes investigated, 13 were detected in the human blastocysts (SPAG9, TMSB10, OXT, POMC, PPY, SCT, LHB, TRH, PRLH, GNRH2, GIP, CCK, and GPHB5) of which four, namely, SPAG9, TMSB10, OXT, and POMC, showed high expression levels. Thirty-two out of the 162 investigated genes coding for human HRs were detected in the human blastocysts, of which NPM1, ATP6AP2, LEPROTL1, and HTR1D showed high expression levels [12, 13, 15–17, 21].

Aneuploidy is common in humans and is the leading cause of all human birth defects as well as miscarriage; errors can arise in meiosis during generation of the oocyte and sperm and in the mitotic divisions of the nascent embryo. A recent study used array-based technology to examine the genome-wide copy number of distinct loci in the cleavage stage human embryos. This study identified several types of chromosomal abnormalities that occurred in human embryos and observed that mosaicism for whole chromosomes (aneuploidies) in one or more blastomeres occurred in more than 80% of embryos [11, 12, 17, 22].

5. Conclusions

Human preimplantation embryos will become an integral and essential part of such endeavors by setting the genetic foundation that determines the course of human development. It is characterized by reprogramming and programming that encompasses fusion of the egg and sperm pronuclei, epigenetic reprogramming, an extensive wave of degradation of maternal transcripts, and activation of the nascent human embryonic genome. The main objective of blastocyst culture was to increase the success rate of in vitro fertilization (IVF) because of better embryo selection after endometrial synchronicity and/or better genomic activation. Metabolism of the blastocyst occurs in two different places: in trophectoderm cells where glucose consumption occurs and half is converted to lactate, whereas glycolysis occurs in ICM. Morphology of the blastocyst depends on the degree of expansion and ICM and TE morphology. This morphological differentiation was thought to represent the developmental capability of the blastocyst. Gene expression during the preimplantation period has identified transcription factors from housekeeping genes, transcription and growth factor genes, sex-determining genes, tissues specifics, novel genes, and genes of unknown functions. Genes unique in human blastocysts included annexins A2 and A3 (ANXA2, ANXA3), gap junction protein alpha 1 (GJPA1), guanosine triphosphate-binding protein 4 (GTPBP4), and adenosine triphosphatase H.–transporting, lysosomal accessory protein 1 (ATP6AP1). The blastocyst-specific genes were associated with oxidative phosphorylation, glycolysis, and sterol metabolism.

Acknowledgements

The authors thank all of team Halim fertility center for their help and support to this book.

Conflict of interest

There is no conflict of interests in this manuscript.

Author details

Hilma Putri Lubis* and Binarwan Halim
Division of Reproductive, Endocrinology, and Infertility, Department of Obstetrics and Gynecology, Faculty of Medicine, Universitas Sumatera Utara, Medan, Indonesia

*Address all correspondence to: hilmaputrilubis@gmail.com

References

[1] Gardner DK, Harvey AJ. Blastocyst metabolism. Reproduction, Fertility, and Development. 2015;**27**:638-654. DOI: 10.1071/RD14421

[2] Gardner DK, Montag M. Human embryo development and assessment of viability. In: Gardner DK, Simon C, editors. Handbook of In Vitro Fertilization. 4th ed. Boca Raton: CRC Press; 2017. pp. 181-204

[3] Gardner DK, Wale PL. Analysis of metabolism to select viable human embryo to transfer. Fertility and Sterility. 2013;**99**:1062-1072. DOI: 10.1016/j.fertnstert.2012.12.004

[4] Jones GM, Trounson AO, Vella PJ, Thouas GA, et al. Glucose metabolism of human morula and blastocyst-stage embryos and its relationship to viability after transfer. Reproductive BioMedicine Online. 2001;**3**(2):124-132

[5] Gardner DK, Wale PL, Collins R, Lane M. Glucose consumption of single post-compaction human embryos is predictive of embryo sex and live birth outcome. Human Reproduction. 2011;**26**:1981-1986. DOI: 10.1093/HUMREP/DER143

[6] Handarson T, Landuyt LV, Jones G. The blastocyst. Human Reproduction. 2012;**27**(S I):i72-i91. DOI: 10.1093/humrep/des230

[7] Carson DD, Bagchi I, De SK, Enders AC. Embryo implantation. Developmental Biology. 2000;**223**:217-237. DOI: 10.1006/dbio.2000.9767

[8] Hardarson T, Caisander C, Sjo¨gren A, Hanson C, Hamberger L, Lundin K. A morphological and chromosomal study of blastocysts developing from morphologically suboptimal human preembryos compared to control blastocysts. Human Reproduction. 2003;**18**:399-407

[9] Alpha Scientists in Reproductive Medicine and ESHRE Special Interest Group of Embryology. The Istanbul consensus workshop on embryo assessment: Proceedings of an expert meeting. Human Reproduction. 2011;**26**:1270-1283

[10] Gardner DK, Schoolcraft WB. In vitro culture of human blastocysts. In: Jansen R, Mortimer D, editors. Toward Reproductive Certainty: Fertility and Genetics Beyond. UK: Parthenon Publishing London; 1999. pp. 378-388

[11] Niakan KK, Han J, Pedersen R, Simon C, Pera AR. Human pre-implantation embryo development. Development. 2012;**139**:829-841. DOI: 10.1242/dev.060426

[12] Pergament E, Fiddler M. The expression of genes in human preimplantation embryos. Prenatal Diagnosis. 1998;**18**:1366-1373

[13] Kakourou G, Jaroudi S, Tulay P, et al. Investigation of gene expression profiles before and after embryonic genome activation and assessment offunctional pathways at the human metaphase II oocyte and blastocyst stage. Fertility and Sterility. 2013;**99**(1):803-814. DOI: 10.1016/j.fertnstert.2012.10.036

[14] Latham KE, Schultz RM. Embryonic genome activation. Frontiers in Bioscience. 2001;**6**:d748-d759

[15] Hamatani T, Daikoku T, Wang H, Matsumoto H, Carter MG, Ko MS, et al. Global gene expression analysis identifies molecular pathways distinguishing blastocyst dormancy and activation. Proceedings of the National Academy of Sciences of the United States of America. 2004;**101**:10326-10331

[16] Hamatani T, Ko M, Yamada M, Kuji N, Mizusawa Y, Shoji M, et al. Global gene expression profiling of

preimplantation embryos. Human Cell. 2006;**19**:98-117

[17] Vanneste E, Voet T, Caignec CL, Ampe M, Konings P, Melotte C, et al. Chromosome instability is common in human cleavage-stage embryos. Nature Medicine. 2009;**15**:577-583

[18] Zhang P, Zucchelli M, Bruce S, Hambiliki F, Stavreus-Evers A, Levkov L, et al. Transcriptome profiling of human preimplantation development. PLoS One. 2009;**4**:e7844

[19] Dobson AT, Raja R, Abeyta MJ, Taylor T, Shen S, Haqq C, et al. The unique transcriptome through day 3 of human preimplantation development. Human Molecular Genetics. 2004;**13**:1461-1470

[20] Eisenberg E, Levanon EY. Human housekeeping genes, revisited. Trends in Genetics. 2013;**1062**:1-6. DOI: 10.1016/j.tig.2013.05.010

[21] Jurisicova A, Casper RF, MacLusky NJ, Librach CL. HLA-G expression during preimplantation human embryo development. Proceedings of the National Academy of Sciences of the United States of America. 1996b;**93**:161-165

[22] Munné S, Lee A, Rosenwaks Z, Grifo J, Cohen J. Diagnosis of major chromosome aneuploidies in human preimplantation embryos. Human Reproduction. 1993;**8**:2185-2191

Chapter 6

Bovine Embryonic Development to Implantation

Loide Valadão, Helena Moreira da Silva and Fernando Moreira da Silva

Abstract

Throughout this chapter, we will express the embryonic development from fertilization, commonly called conception, to the implantation. It is well documented that preimplantation is considered a critical period for embryo development in ruminants, in which high pregnancy loss occurs; in fact, several authors point out that 50–75% of blastocysts fail to implant. The high rate of implantation failure is one reason why pregnancy typically requires on average two ovulation cycles to achieve. Events involved in the embryo growth and survival are directly or indirectly related to cytokines, steroids, metabolites, and growth factors. When one of these compounds fails, it normally leads to the death of the embryo or fetus. As known, the period required for full development of a fetus in utero is referred to as gestation, and it is commonly subdivided into two distinct periods. The first 2 weeks of prenatal development are referred to as the pre-embryonic stage. By the end of the embryonic period, all of the organ systems are structured in rudimentary form, and the embryo shifts to the fetus from the ninth week of gestation until birth.

Keywords: bovine, oocyte, fertilization, embryonic development implantation

1. Introduction

The reproductive system of the bovine female includes several organs such as ovaries, genital pathways or tubular portion that surround the oviducts, uterus, vagina, and vulva, the attached glands, embryonic vestiges, blood vessels, and nerves. The ovaries have two differentiated portions: a medullary zone formed by connective tissue, fibroelastic and vessels (arteries, veins, and lymphatics), and nerves, all together responsible for the conservation and nutrition of the organ. The other portion is the cortical zone, which is surrounded by the germinal epithelium and the tunica albuginea within it. The follicles and corpora lutea in their different stages of development and regression are located in this last portion. In adult females, this structure of the cortical zone undergoes cyclical changes according to the regulation of the sexual cycle or of pregnancy. The female sexual organs include two functions essential to the reproduction of females, a gametogenic function, composed by folliculogenesis and oogenesis, and an endocrine function in which the main produced hormones are estrogen, progesterone, and relaxin. The ovary of the cow or heifer, relatively to its weight is small when compared to other species, has an ovoid shape and varies in size and contour at each cycle due to the projection of follicles and corpus lutea on its surface (**Figure 1**).

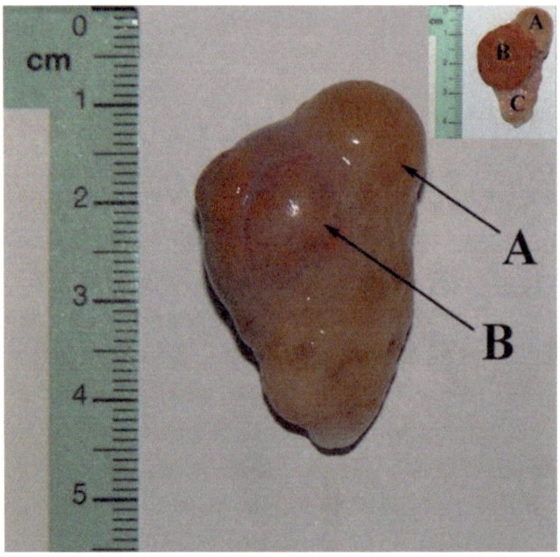

Figure 1.
The ovary where the following can be observed: A follicle (A) and a corpus luteum (B). In the upper right corner, these ovarian structures are emphasized.

Its weight ranges from 3 to 20 g and can reach 37 mm in length. In the cortical area of the ovaries, structures called follicles are present, which cyclically enter the growth phase. On average, if cow or heifer is not pregnant, a follicle grows and ovulates every 21 days. When follicles reach maturation, they rupture and release the oocyte within. The primordial follicle is an oocyte surrounded by a single layer of low follicular cells. When these cells multiply by mitosis, this is called the secondary follicle. When it reaches its maximum development, it is called the vesicular, mature, or antrum follicle. Follicular development is observed in the fetal period, in prepubescent heifers, heifers, and cyclic cows and during gestation. The oocytes are conceived from germ cells that originate the female sex cells, which contain in their cytoplasm ribosomes, mitochondria, glycogen granules, large lipid droplets and endoplasmic reticulum, and poorly developed Golgi complex. During oocyte growth, changes in the distribution, number, and size of cytoplasmic organelles occur [1]. The oocyte is surrounded by the zona pellucida (**Figure 2**), which is a dense membrane with multiple functions, being primordial for the normal development of the follicle [2].

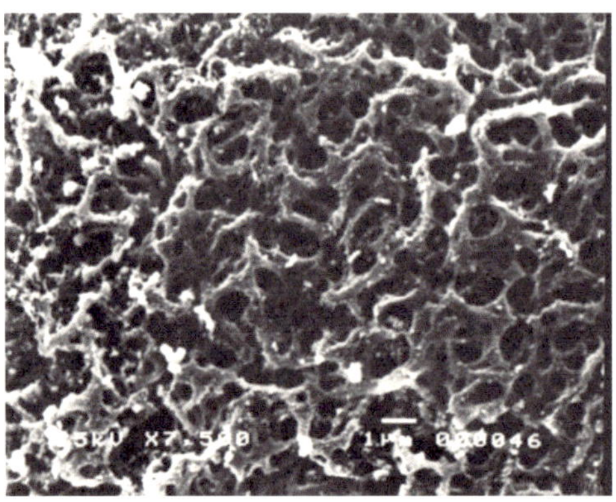

Figure 2.
Fine detail of a bovine oocyte zone pellucida captured by transmission electron microscopy. The bar represents 1 μm.

2. Oocyte maturation and ovulation

During the evolution of the oocyte, the nucleus that had entered the prophase of the first meiotic division will support the reductive divisions. Two daughter cells appear that contain half of the chromosome load in the first division, where each of the cells gets a large part of the cytoplasm, called the secondary oocyte. The smaller one is called the first polar body. Throughout the second meiotic division, the secondary oocyte divides into two (ovoid and second polar body). The corpus luteum is an endocrine gland that occurs by cycles in the ovary of females and has a short secretory activity during the sexual cycle. In the bovine species, it has an ovoid or spherical shape. Its main function is the production of progesterone, which is responsible for the preparation of the endometrium and the blastocyst for implantation. According to Gordon [3], it takes 11 days for the corpus luteum to develop and reach a 4 g weight in a female of beef cattle; in a female of milk breed, its weight is higher. The fast growth of the yellow body in the first phase of the ovulatory cycle occurs until the tenth day.

The infundibulum is a funnel-shaped tube that encloses the ovary during the ovulation. It serves to capture oocytes and channels them to the oviduct, where fertilization occurs in the presence of viable spermatozoa [4]. Finally, the uterus is a muscular, cavitary, pelvic abdominal organ and with great capacity of dilation and displacement to welcome the development of the embryo. This organ is divided into three parts, uterine horns and posteriorly, through the cranial orifice of the cervical canal, cervix which is the caudal portion of the uterus with a well-individualized structure due to its thick wall, constricted light and full of protrusions and recesses, the cervical rings [1]. The body of the cow's uterus is short and undeveloped. Its size varies with age and number of deliveries and can reach 5 cm in length. It has several functions like assisting the transport of the spermatozoa to the oviduct and helping in the expulsion of the newborn. In this organ the placenta that will allow nutrition and protection to the fetus also develops [4]. The cervix is a unique structure within the reproductive apparatus of the cow. It has thick walls and attaches the vagina to the uterus. Its main function is to protect the uterus from the external environment.

The vagina is a copulatory organ that has a thin, elastic wall that allows its distension during mating and delivery. It serves as a free passage for the calf at the time of its expulsion.

Folliculogenesis begins with the formation of primordial follicles, progressing to primary, secondary, tertiary, and preovulatory, and ends with the ovulation of a mature oocyte (**Figure 3**).

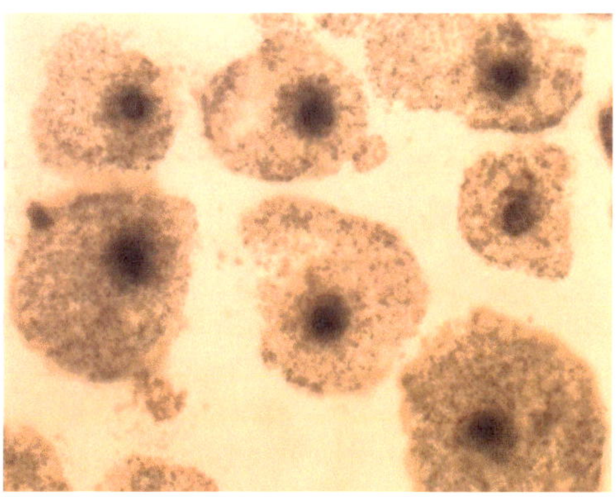

Figure 3.
Bovine typical oocyte's aspect after maturation.

That is a process of follicular formation, growth, and maturation involving the proliferation and differentiation of cells [2]. These cycles start when heifer attains puberty, but the development of oocytes and follicles begins in the mother's uterus before the calving. Primordial germ cells proliferate by mitosis to form primary oocytes; the first meiotic prophase starts between days 75 and 80 of pregnancy [5]. At the diplotene stage of meiosis (around day 170), a primordial follicle forms; the oocyte is delimited by a single layer of 4–8 pre-granulosa cells. Then, these oocytes remain in the resting phase until they are stimulated to grow [6] until ovulation or became an atresic follicle. Factors regulating formation of primordial follicles are not well known [7]. Russe [8] postulated that primordial, primary, and secondary follicles appear in the fetal ovary on days 90, 140, and 210, respectively. A secondary follicle is characterized by the addition of a second layer of granulosa cells [9], the initial deposition of zona pellucida material, formation of cortical granules within the oocyte cytoplasm, onset of oocyte RNA synthesis [10], and gonadotrophin responsiveness [7]. The transition to the tertiary follicle includes development of the theca interna and externa, the basal lamina, and cumulus cells, as well as the formation of a fluid-filled antral cavity [9]. At this stage, follicles can attain a tremendous size being impaired only by the availability of FSH, as at this time they are dependent on. The oocyte reaches the stage of metaphase II, just before ovulation. Only if the oocyte reaches this meiosis stage it can be able to be fertilized.

3. Oocyte fertilization

Fertilization is a complex sequence of events that begins with the contact of a spermatozoid with an oocyte and culminates with the mixture of the maternal and paternal chromosomes in the metaphase of the first mitotic division of the embryo. The union of the male gametes with the female gametes involves several phases. Firstly, the passage of the sperm through the radiata corona that surrounds the zona pellucida of the oocyte [11]. The movements of the spermatozoa tail are important for its penetration into the radiata corona. The most important phase of the initiation of fertilization involves the penetration of the surrounding zona pellucida to the oocyte. Then, the fusion of the plasma membranes of the oocyte and the spermatozoid occurs in which the head and tail of the same penetrate the cytoplasm of the oocyte, leaving the plasma membrane behind. After entering the spermatozoa, the oocyte that was in the metaphase of the second meiotic division completes this division, and completing this division forms a mature oocyte and a second polar body. Within the cytoplasm of the oocyte, the nucleus of the sperm increases in size, forming the male pronucleus [12]. The membranes of the pronucleus dissolve and the chromosomes condense and prepare to mitotic cell division, ending up to 24 h after ovulation [13]. Pronuclear fusion and mitosis are most easily seen with transparent eggs, with low-power microscopic magnification that the originally eccentric pronucleus moves to the center of the egg at about 20–30 min after fertilization and that the nuclear envelope disappears as the egg enters late prophase.

The first provided a description of bovine ovulated oocytes and two-cell stage embryos which was made by Hartmen and collaborators in 1931 [14], but only 15 years later, a more detailed description of developmental stages, from the unfertilized oocyte to the blastocyst, was reported by Hamilton and Laing [15]. Concerning the activation of embryonic genome, the zygote and early cleavage-stage embryo are thought to be controlled maternally hereditary by mRNA molecules until genomic activation occurs. The transition from oogenetic to embryonic genomic activation (EGA) is called the maternal-to-embryonic transition (MET) [16] and allows further embryogenesis to become dependent on the expression of the embryonic genome [17, 18]. In the bovine, the onset of MET occurs at the 8- to 16-cell stage. However, it was suggested that the onset of MET may be controlled temporally (i.e., at a time after fertilization) rather than at a developmental stage, as minor transcriptional activity was detected as early as the pronuclear stage after in vitro fertilization (reviewed by [19]).

In cattle, the gestation has a duration of approximately 282 days, being divided in three stages. In a first phase, the formation of the zygote occurs, and the implantation of the embryo begins. Then, in the second stage, the onset of trophoectodermal adhesion to the endometrium occurs, and the culmination of the embryonic differentiation period occurs when the onset of fetal bone mineralization occurs. The last stage is called the fetal phase that is between the beginning of fetal bone mineralization and moment of the expulsion of the fetus.

4. Embryo development

In the oviduct, after fertilization, while the one-cell embryos are projected toward the uterus by peristalsis and beating cilia, the zygotes undergo five or six rapid mitotic cell divisions, not increasing, however, the total volume of the conceptus. The cleavage of the zygote is defined as being repeated mitotic divisions of the zygote, which leads to a rapid increase in the number of cells (blastomeres). These are decreasing in size with each division of the cleavage. The zygote first divides into two blastomeres, and then these two cells divide into four blastomeres, eight blastomeres, and so on (**Figure 4**). This division occurs about 30 h after fertilization, followed by other divisions, forming progressively smaller blastomeres [20]. Up to the eight-cell stage, these form a cluster. After the third cleavage, the blastomeres maximize their contact with each other, giving rise to a compact cluster of cells, called compaction. Three days after the fertilization approximately, the cells of the compacted embryonic structure divide again to form 16 cells (morula). As morula embryo continues growing, these blastomeres will divide into two kinds of cells. The inner cell mass, that is, the inner cells of the morula, which will give birth to the embryo tissues, and the surrounding cells create the external cell mass that will contribute to the formation of the placenta [13]. Then once inside the uterus (about 4–5 days after fertilization), the conceptus floats freely for several more days, creating a ball of approximately 100 cells and consuming nutritive endometrial secretions called uterine milk while the uterine lining thickens, and the conceptus is referred to as a blastocyst.

Within this structure, a small amount of cells forms an inner cell mass, which will become the embryo and then the fetus. The other cells form the outer shell are called trophoblasts (trophe = "to feed" or "to nourish") and then will develop into the chorionic sac and the fetal portion of the placenta (the organ of nutrient, waste,

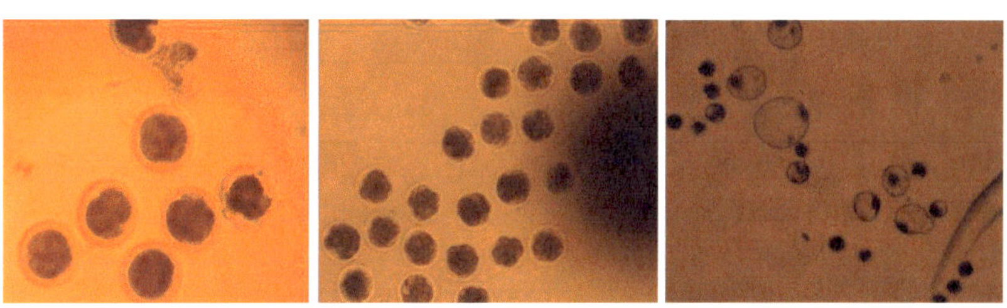

Figure 4.
Bovine oocytes after fertilization: on day 2 between two and four cells (on the left side), on day 6 as the morula stage (on the center), and on day 9 as blastocysts (on the right side).

and gas exchange between mother and the developing offspring). This mother/embryo dialog induces dynamic changes in the uterine epithelia, tightly regulated by steroid hormones, cytokines, and growth factors, which establish uterine receptivity toward the developing conceptus. The inner mass of embryonic cells is totipotent during this stage, meaning that each cell has the potential to differentiate into any cell type in the body. In a process called "hatching," the conceptus breaks free of the zona pellucida and the implantation begins. The blastocyst typically implants in the fundus of the uterus or on the posterior wall. At this time the trophoblast secretes pregnancy serum protein B (PSPB or PAG), a hormone that directs the corpus luteum to survive, enlarge, and continue producing progesterone and estrogen to suppress menses, as well as to create an environment suitable for the developing embryo. Studies developed in our department clearly showed that PAG/PSPB increases from the beginning to the end of pregnancy, reaching its maximum in the calving day [21, 22].

The cells of the inner cell mass are now an embryoblast, which are in a pole, and the cells of the outer cell mass are called trophoblast, which flatten and form the epithelial wall of the blastocyst. At this stage the embryo separates from the zona pellucida allowing the beginning of the implantation. In bovine, although the blastocyst is formed several days after fertilization, placentation starts on day 21, beginning then the implantation. The uterus upon implantation is in the secretory phase; the blastocyst is implanted in the endometrium along the anterior or posterior wall [23]. The trophoblast differentiates into a single nucleus of mitotically active cells, called cytotrophoblast, and a rapidly expanding multinucleated mass, syncytiotrophoblast, which causes erosion of maternal tissues. On the ninth day, gaps are formed in the syncytiotrophoblast. Subsequently, the maternal sinusoids are eroded by the syncytiotrophoblast, the mother's blood passes into the lacunar network, and at the end of the second week, the primitive uteroplacental circulation begins. During this time, the blastocyst is perfectly implanted and consolidated. The embryoblast is differentiated into epiblast and hypoblast, which form the bilaminar disk. Amnioblasts are lining the amniotic cavity superiorly to the epiblast layer. In turn, the hypoblast cells are continuous with the exocoelomic membrane, and together they surround the primitive yolk sac. The amniotic cavity and the yolk sac are formed from the primitive extra-embryonic mesoderm with the onset of somatopleure and splanchnopleure.

During the third week, gastrulation occurs which is the process by which the bilaminar embryonic disk is converted into a trilaminar embryonic disk (beginning of morphogenesis). Gastrulation begins with the appearance of the primitive line where the primitive node is at its cephalic end. Epiblast cells in the knot and primitive line are invaginated to form new leaflets (endoderm and mesoderm). At the end of the third week, the three basic germ leaflets in the cephalic region (ectoderm, mesoderm, and endoderm) are already demonstrated [13]. The ectoderm gives rise to organs and structures that maintain contact with the exterior, central nervous system, peripheral nervous system, pituitary gland, mammary glands, sweat glands, and tooth enamel. By the end of the fourth week, there is the production of these germ leaflets in the more caudal areas of the embryo. Differentiation of tissues, extra-embryonic membranes, and organs begins (**Figure 5**).

The trophoblast progresses rapidly. The primary villi obtain a mesenchymal core, and the small capillaries originate. When these villous capillaries come in contact with capillaries on the chorionic plaque and the attachment pedicle, the villous system is ready to provide the embryo with nutrients and oxygen [11]. During this time, embryo-maternal crosstalk remains one of the most challenging subjects in reproductive biology. The decoding of embryo-maternal interactions may allow the development of new therapeutic strategies to enhance embryonic survival,

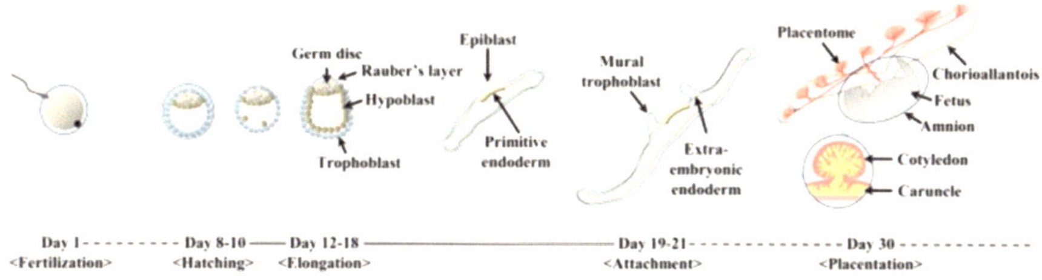

Figure 5.
Schematic development of a bovine embryo from fertilization to day 30 (adapted from [23]).

which would have a major impact in cattle reproductive efficiency and profitability of modern cattle industry providing relevant advancements in our knowledge of the determinants of normal and abnormal deviations of health.

5. Strategies to improve embryo survival

Several strategies have been designed to enhance embryo survival. Due to its unequivocal role in pregnancy establishment and maintenance, P4-based strategies have received great attention from both researchers and practitioners. Strategies designed to increase post-ovulatory peripheral concentrations of P4 include increasing peripheral levels of P4 or manipulating nutrition either to decrease plasma concentrations of E2 or inhibiting the PGF2α-synthesizing enzymatic machinery in the endometrium during the critical period [24, 25]. Hormonal manipulations to increase P4 include direct P4 supplementation [26] and administration of gonadotrophin-releasing hormone (GnRH; [27]), bovine somatotropin (BST; [28]), equine chorionic gonadotrophin (eCG; [29]), and human chorionic gonadotrophin (hCG; [30]).

6. Fetal period

The fetal period begins 9 weeks after fertilization and ends at birth. It is characterized by being a period of rapid body growth and maturation of organs and systems. At first, the fetus increases its length more rapidly than it gains weight. In the third trimester of gestation, the length increases slowly increasing rapidly in weight. The energy requirements of the fetus increase from the third trimester of gestation. Fetus size varies according to genetic factors, such as race, fetus phenotype, and other environmental factors, such as the mother's age, nutrition, and management.

7. Conclusion

Embryonic development has fascinated scientists and philosophers from ancient culture to the present day. Once fertilized, the zygote travels down the fallopian tube and mitotically divides many times to form a droplet of cells called a blastocyst. The blastocyst consists of an inner mass that develops into the embryo, while the outer layer develops into tissue that nourishes and protects the embryo. The blastocyst attaches onto the wall of the uterus and receives nourishment through the mother's blood. The major systems structures of the calf develop during the embryonic period in a process called differentiation. During this stage, kidney, brain, spinal cord, nerve, heart, and blood cells start to develop, and the gastrointestinal tract begins to form. Despite years of dedicated research, much still remains to be discovered on the formation of gametes (the sex cells), fertilization, and the subsequent development of the embryo.

Acknowledgements

This project was financed in 85% by FEDER and in 15% with regional funds through the Programa Operacional Açores 2020 (Operational Program Azores 2020), in scope of the project "BEMAP-ET - ACORES-01-0145-FEDER-000026."

Conflict of interest

The authors declare, for all legal purposes, the absence of any conflict of interest related to this paper.

Author details

Loide Valadão, Helena Moreira da Silva and Fernando Moreira da Silva*
Faculty of Agrarian Sciences and Environment, CITA-A (Research Centre for Agricultural and Environmental Sciences and Technology of the Azores), Animal Reproduction, University of the Azores, Angra do Heroismo, Portugal

*Address all correspondence to: joaquim.fm.silva@uac.pt

References

[1] Antunes G, Marques A, Santos P, Chaveiro A, Moreira da Silva F. 2008. Atlas do ovócito e do embrião Bovino–Breves noções da fisiologia da reprodução em bovinos. Edited by F. Moreira da Silva-Principia-Lisbon, Portugal. (120 pp)

[2] Adona PR, Monzani PS, Guemra S, Miranda MS, Ohashi OM. Oogenesis and folliculogenesis in mammals. UNOPAR Científica. Ciências Biológicas e da Saúde. 2012;**15**(3):245-250

[3] Gordon I. Laboratory Production of Cattle Embryos. 2nd ed. Washington: Cabi Publishing; 2013. 548p

[4] Lourenço JCX. Efeito do choque térmico na maturação nuclear e avaliação da expressão genética em ovócitos de bovino [MSc thesis]. University of the Azores; 2016. 56p

[5] Erickson BH. Development and senescence of the post-natal bovine ovary. Journal of Animal Science. 1966;**25**:800-805

[6] Erickson BH. Development and radio-response of the prenatal bovine ovary. Journal of Reproduction and Fertility. 1966;**11**:97-105

[7] Fair T. Follicular oocyte growth and acquisition of developmental competence. Animal Reproduction Science. 2003;**78**:203-216

[8] Russe I. Oogenesis in cattle and sheep. Bibliotheca Anatomica. 1983;**24**:77-92

[9] Driancourt MA. Follicular dynamics in sheep and cattle. Theriogenology. 1991;**35**:55-68

[10] Fair T, Hulshof SCJ, Hyttel P, Boland M, Greve T. Bovine oocyte ultrastructure in primordial to tertiary follicles. Anatomy and Embryology. 1997;**195**:327-336

[11] Sadler TW. Langman embriologia médica. 7th ed. Guanabara Koogan-São Paulo-Brasil; 2005. 320p

[12] Lee JW, Tian XC, Yang X. Failure of male pronucleus formation is the major cause of lack of fertilization and embryo development in pig oocytes subjected to intracytoplasmic sperm injection. Biology of Reproduction. 2003;**68**(4):1341-1347

[13] Sadler TW. Langman embriologia médica. 9th ed. Guanabara Koogan-São Paulo-Brasil; 2005. 347p

[14] Hartmen CG, Lewis WH, Miller FW, Swett WW. First findings of tubal ova in the cow, together with notes on oestrus. The Anatomical Record. 1931;**48**:267-275

[15] Hamilton WJ, Laing JA. Development of the egg of the cow up to the stage of blastocyst formation. Journal of Anatomy. 1946;**80**:194-204

[16] Telford NA, Watson AJ, Schultz GA. Transition from maternal to embryonic control in early mammalian development: A comparison of several species. Molecular Reproduction and Development. 1990;**26**:90-100

[17] Kanka J. Gene expression and chromatin structure in the preimplantation embryo. Theriogenology. 2003;**59**:3-19

[18] Walser CB, Lipshitz HD. Transcript clearance during the maternal-to-zygotic transition. Current Opinion in Genetics and Development. 2011;**21**:431-443

[19] Kanka J, Nemcova L, Toralova T, Vodickova-Kepkova K, Vodicka P, Jeseta M, et al. Association of the transcription profile of bovine oocytes and embryos with developmental potential. Animal Reproduction Science. 2012;**134**(1-2):29-35

[20] Moore KL, Persaud TVN. Embriologia básica. 5th ed. Guanabara Koogan-São Paulo-Brasil; 2000. 453p

[21] Metelo R, Moreira da Silva F, Beckers JF. Determination of pregnancy-associated glycoprotein (bPAG) in cow's milk. In: 23rd World Buitics Congress. 2004. p. 75

[22] Metelo R, Sulon J, Moreira da Silva F, Beckers JF. Preliminary results for measuring bovine PAG in milk simples. 7ème Journée de Rencontre Bioforum, BioLiège, Association des Biotechnologistes Liégeois, Liège, 3 May 2002. p. 32

[23] Bai H, Sakurai T, Godkin JD, Imakawa K. Expression and potential role of GATA factors in trophoblast development. Journal of Reproduction and Development. 2013;**59**(1):1-6

[24] Binelli M, Thatcher WW, Mattos R, Baruselli PS. Antiluteolytic strategies to improve fertility in cattle. Theriogenology. 2015;**6**:1451-1463

[25] Inskeep EK. Preovulatory, postovulatory, and postmaternal recognition effects of concentrations of progesterone on embryonic survival in the cow. Journal of Animal Science. 2004;**82**(E):E24-E39

[26] Stevenson JS, Portaluppi MA, Tenhouse DE, Lloyd A, Eborn DR, Kacuba S, et al. Interventions after artificial insemination: Conception rates, pregnancy survival, and ovarian responses to gonadotropin-releasing hormone, human chorionic gonadotropin, and progesterone. Journal of Dairy Science. 2007;**90**(1):331-340

[27] Pursley JR, Martins JP. Impact of circulating concentrations of progesterone and antral age of the ovulatory follicle on fertility of high-producing lactating dairy cows. Reproduction, Fertility, and Development. 2011;**24**(1):267-271

[28] Moreira F, Badinga L, Burnley C, Thatcher WW. Bovine somatotropin increases embryonic development in superovulated cows and improves post-transfer pregnancy rates when given to lactating recipient cows. Theriogenology. 2002;**57**:1371-1387

[29] Bartolome JA, Wallace SP, de la Sota RL, Thatcher WW. The effect of administering equine chorionic gonadotropin (eCG) and human chorionic gonadotropin (hCG) post artificial insemination on fertility of lactating dairy cows. Theriogenology. 2012;**78**(5):1110-1116

[30] De Rensis F, López-Gatius F, García-Ispierto I, Techakumpu M. Clinical use of human chorionic gonadotrophin in dairy cows: An update. Theriogenology. 2010;**73**(8):1001-1008

Chapter 7

The Role of Neuroendocrine in Embryo Implantation

Fenting Liu and Rong Li

Abstract

Neuroendocrine integration, an integration of the nervous system and endocrine system as its name implies, plays a critical role in the reproductive system. However, less progress has been made in the particular effects of neuroendocrine on embryo implantation. Recently, some significant knowledges have been gained on the regulation of neuroendocrine in embryo implantation. This chapter will summarize the current state of knowledges about the impaction of neuroendocrine on embryo implantation and discuss potential strategy to get higher pregnancy rate and to reduce recurrent implantation failure (RIF) possibility through modulating the neuroendocrine systems.

Keywords: neuroendocrine systems, embryo implantation, recurrent implantation failure, IVF-ET

1. Introduction

The success of mammalian pregnancy is mostly due to the smoothly embryo implantation into the maternal endometrium/decidua, which is a finely regulated process and requires the adaptation of maternal function to the needs of developing fetus. Human embryo implantation is a complex series of events involving blastocyst attachment, adhesion, and invasion into the endometrial tissue. Under normal circumstances, in order to ensure the consistency of this series, the blastocyst-stage embryo and the uterine endometrium must be collaborated during the "window of implantation" [1]. It has been long established that neuroendocrine is indispensable for mammalian reproduction [2], in which the neuroendocrine cell can synthesize and release various hormones into gonadal organ after receiving neuronal signal. Notably, the hypothalamus is the metronome of reproduction, and its main function is to receive neural signals from the brain and transform these neural signals into an endocrine output, the pulsatile release of GnRH, and other related factors. The pituitary gland, as a link between the brain and other neuroendocrine-related organs, is divided into two lobes. For the anterior lobe, it is related to the regulation of the hypothalamic-pituitary-gonadal axis (HPG axis), hypothalamic-pituitary-thyroid axis (HPT axis), and hypothalamic-pituitary-adrenal axis (HPA axis). For the posterior lobe, it is mainly about the regulation of the hypothalamic-neurohypophysis system [3]. Therefore, the description of an importance of the neuroendocrine to implantation from the aspects above is an enormous and necessary work.

Infertility affects millions of couples worldwide and its treatment has progressed immensely. As one of the most prevalent approaches of treating infertility, in vitro fertilization and embryo transfer (IVF-ET) is always confronted with recurrent implantation failure [4], which is in the means of the situation when the transferred embryo repeatedly, failed to implant after IVF-ET [5]. A strong association between pregnancy rate following IVF-ET and recurrent implantation failure has been investigated [4], but less studies mention directly about the role of neuroendocrine in recurrent implantation failure. A thorough understanding of the processes governing human embryo implantation would be of significant benefit for the treatment of infertility. Hence, this review provides a summary of current empirical researches on the impacts of neuroendocrine aspects in implantation so that we more understand the maternal environment at the time of embryo implantation and might optimize it by altering neuroendocrine regulation to increase the success rate after IVF-ET.

2. Hypothalamic-pituitary-gonadal axis

An integrated hypothalamic-pituitary-gonadal axis with several main actors including the gonadotropin-releasing hormone (GnRH), the gonadotropins (luteinizing hormone (LH) and follicular-stimulating hormone (FSH)), and the gonadal hormones are recognized as a key mechanism on human reproduction [6]. Hypothalamic gonadotropin-releasing hormone, as a crucial regulator of the HPG axis, with characteristic pulsatile secretion pattern, plays a dominant role in the endocrine control of reproduction and its possible effects on implantation by regulating downstream hormones which have been widely concerned so far [7]. Two GnRH molecules termed GnRH I (default as GnRH) and GnRH isoform II (GnRH II) can be found in humans, and both of them play an important role during the implantation period as shown in **Figure 1** [6, 8].

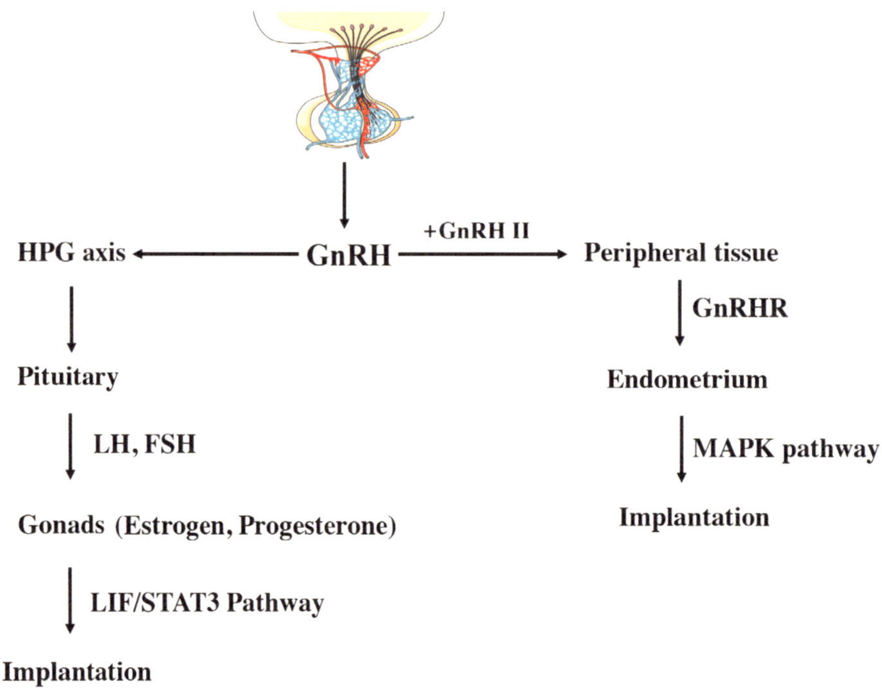

Figure 1.
Schematic of the HPG axis functions in implantation.

2.1 GnRH functions in implantation via the pituitary-gonadal axis

In the HPG axis, after releasing from the hypothalamus in a pulsatile manner, GnRH then binds to GnRH receptors (GnRHRs) on the pituitary gland, in response, that LH and FSH are synthesized and secreted in pulse by the pituitary to match the GnRH signal. Subsequently steroid hormones including progesterone and estrogen are released from the gonads and form a loop by exerting a positive or a negative feedback effect on GnRH releasing and gonadotropin [8]. Although it has been reported that human type II receptor for GnRH II shows specific expression of the receptor in the anterior pituitary and it also has been suggested that these receptors might act together to regulate the biosynthesis and secretion of both LH and FSH, further investigation should be completed [9, 10]. Thus here, we focus on the functions of GnRH in implantation via the pituitary-gonadal axis. Since natural GnRH has a short half-life, several GnRH synthetic analogues have been developed including agonists and antagonists, which can be used to stimulate or block, respectively, the pituitary-gonadal axis in an assisted reproductive technology (ART), particularly often applied to prevent premature LH surge [11]. In women undergoing IVF, GnRH agonist may improve the luteal phase support, used to trigger the final oocyte maturation and to improve implantation and live birth rates [12]. Although the effects of embryo implantation are still controversial, both of them are thought to tightly correspond to the pituitary-gonadal axis and eventually result in the fluctuation of the estrogen and progesterone level [6, 11].

Estrogen and progesterone regulate uterine cell proliferation and are necessary for the changes in both the blastocyst and uterine epithelium for successful adhesion, so an imbalance between estrogen and progesterone during the luteal phase may lead to implantation defects [13]. Thus, it is quite clear that a deep understanding of the action of estrogen and progesterone on the human endometrium will allow a clear insight into the mechanism of determining endometrial receptivity in embryo implantation.

So far, the molecular mechanism of estrogen regulation of maternal uterus in implantation remains unclear. Some studies implicated that estrogen was not essential for embryo implantation due to its receptor disappearance at the time of implantation [14, 15]. However, some studies believed that only after sufficient exposure to estrogen could progesterone exposure drive the endometrial receptivity to embryo implantation in a brief period [16, 17]. In addition, it has been proven that early growth response 1 (Egr1) as the downstream target is regulated by estrogen expression via leukemia inhibitory factor-signal transducer and activator of transcription 3 (LIF-STAT3) signaling pathway in the uterus of a mouse, and it further regulates stromal cell decidualization by regulating Wnt4 [18]. Furthermore, some studies suggested that estrogen was a trigger to close the window of implantation via insulin-like growth factor 1 pathway and made the endometrium "receptive" for blastocyst implantation [19, 20].

Progesterone production reaches its peak during the mid-luteal phase of the cycle, and this is the time when the secretory endometrium is appropriately prepared for the implantation of an embryo [8]. During the luteal phase, progesterone is produced, in turn stimulating the proliferation of the lining of the uterus to prepare for implantation by blocking the production of matrix metalloproteinase (MMP) and stimulating the production of tissue factor (TF) and plasminogen activator inhibitor 1 (PAI-1) [21, 22]. The phenomenon that a luteal phase support with progesterone can improve the implantation and pregnancy rates indicates lower progesterone and lower implantation [23, 24]. A review by Yoshinaga further confirms that progesterone is also an indispensable factor for successful implantation and pregnancy maintenance [19].

2.2 GnRH functions in implantation via peripheral reproductive tissue

The expression of GnRH/GnRH receptor (GnRHR) system and GnRH II in the female reproductive tissues has been widely reported. Therefore, in addition to its well-known function on the HPG axis, GnRH and GnRH II may also regulate extrapituitary reproductive tissues through the local GnRHRs [24]. Both GnRH and GnRH II have a dynamic pattern during the process of implantation; they may regulate the procedure of trophoblast local invasion and embryo implantation through the regulation of the proteolytic degradation of the extracellular matrix of the endometrial stroma and the motility of decidua endometrial stromal cells [6]. During the luteal phase of the menstrual cycle, high levels of both GnRH and GnRHR are expressed in the endometrium; thus the blastocyst will prefer to attach the endometrial epithelial surface and go through implantation [5, 7]. In mammals, the distribution of GnRH II is more wide in peripheral tissue than that of GnRH I, which hypothesized that GnRH II has extra functions and a possible regulator in endometrial environment [9]. Huang et al. found that GnRH II could directly regulate the behavior of endometrial cells. An embryo implantation failure may be due to the dysfunction of human decidual endometrial stromal cell motility via different pathways [25]. The hallmark events of implantation are represented by tissue remodeling and angiogenesis, which are regulated by the activity of MMPs and tissue inhibitors of MMPs (TIMPs) [26]. It has been demonstrated that GnRH II may contribute to the regulation of the cell motility of decidual endometrial stromal cells via the binding of GnRH-IRs, in turn stimulating the expression of MAPK-mediated proteinases MMP-2 and MMP-9, which specifically degrade the basement membrane and then facilitate the invasion and migration of decidual endometrial stromal cells [6].

Given the evidence above, no matter via the GnRHR in the pituitary-gonadal axis or via GnRHR in peripheral reproductive tissue, both pathways of GnRH functions on implantation are potential candidate therapeutic targets for improving the embryo implantation rate in the treatment of infertility.

3. Hypothalamus-pituitary-adrenal axis

In addition to the well-established role of the HPG axis in implantation and infertility, the role of the hypothalamic-pituitary-adrenal axis (HPA axis) in the reproductive tract also cannot be neglected. A hormone cycle also exists in the HPA axis. After receiving neuronal signals, the corticotropin-releasing hormone (CRH) secreted from the hypothalamus transports to function in the pituitary gland to release adrenocorticotropic hormone (ACTH) and subsequently acts on the adrenal cortex to produce glucocorticoid (GC) hormones (mainly cortisol in humans). Eventually, the glucocorticoid hormones will act back on the hypothalamus and pituitary (to suppress CRH and ACTH production) in a negative feedback cycle [3]. The hormone within the HPA axis can act at different levels of the HPG axis as well as the uterus and other peripheral tissues; therefore we will discuss it in the following part, respectively.

3.1 CRH functions in implantation

CRH is taking the lead in the HPA axis, and its expression is mediated by its membrane receptors including CRH-R1 and CRH-R2 [27]. According to the research, upregulating gal-1 expression by acting through the CRHR1 in Ishikawa cell line and macrophages indeed indicates that CRH plays a critical role in implantation [28]. CRH has tremendous effects on implantation since it can impact the HPG axis at different levels. In mammals, numerous GnRH-containing neurons in the hypothalamus have been found to express both CRH receptors (CRH-R1, CRH-R2) which can exert an estradiol-dependent effect of directly influencing GnRH release in mice and rats, leading to a comparable change in serum LH levels, and eventually contribute to the difference of response during implantation procedure [29].

Besides, CRH serving as an autocrine and paracrine modulator is expressed in peripheral tissue of the female reproductive system, including the endometrium [30]. Early pregnancy, containing a higher concentration of CRH in the endometrium of a rat and killing activated T lymphocytes, can promote implantation and maintain pregnancy [31]. Furthermore, CRH can downregulate the expression of carcinoembryonic antigen-related cell adhesion molecule 1 (CEACAM1) by extravillous trophoblast cells, thereby controlling proper trophoblast invasion during implantation [32].

3.2 ACTH functions in implantation

Besides the downstream effects from CRH, ACTH also has its certain effects in implantation, though fewer studies have been investigated. Similar to CRH, chronic ACTH stimulation also impacts on the HPG axis by inhibiting LH secretion to impair the procedure of implantation. In the contrary, acute ACTH treatment may result in a rapid increase of progesterone which will lead to a positive feedback and induce the elevation of LH and FSH within the HPG axis [33]. A reference implied that exogenous ACTH produced postponed implantation effects and resulted in the high incidence of miscarriage and embryonic resorption [34]. However, further investigation should be performed.

3.3 Glucocorticoid functions in implantation

Glucocorticoid (GC) is a measurement of stress and leads to well-characterized profound reproduction function by suppressing the HPG axis and influencing the peripheral tissue [35]. Some studies indicated that maintaining the administration of glucocorticoids could improve pregnancy rates and outcomes both in animals and human beings [36, 37]. Therefore, to elucidate the role of glucocorticoids in implantation, the following two dimensions will be depicted.

3.3.1 Via the HPG axis

As a pivotal hormone in the HPA axis, GC has been demonstrated with the function of decreasing the release of GnRH from the hypothalamus, both directly and indirectly inhibiting GnRH pulses or inhibiting upstream regulators of GnRH release, in turn exerting direct effects on the anterior pituitary of the release of the gonadotropins, eventually influencing the steroid hormones from gonads [38].

GnRH-containing neurons also express glucocorticoid receptors (GRs) and have an effect of directly inhibiting GnRH release in mice and rats, leading to a decrease of serum LH [39]. Besides, evidences showed that chronic corticosterone (CORT) treatment could inhibit directly GnRH release in the hypothalamus and influence on implantation and reproduction [29, 40]. Another method is via modulating the hormones upstream of GnRH, mainly including kisspeptin (KISS1) and RFamide-related peptide-3 (RFRP-3) [41]. Both of these two hormones express GRs, implying that they could potentially respond to GC and suppress the release of GnRH, leading to the fluctuation of LH and FSH from the pituitary [42].

In addition to the secondary signaling effects on the pituitary, glucocorticoid can directly inhibit its secretion by different mechanisms at the level of the pituitary, including modulating the sensitivity of the pituitary to changes in GnRH secretion and further decreasing the synthesis and secretion of LH and FSH from the pituitary [43]. However, a study showed that the effects of glucocorticoid directly on the pituitary in secretion and synthesis were highly variable [44]; thereby further studies should be performed in this field.

The gonads, as the lowest level in the HPG axis, are another crucial component for glucocorticoids to regulate, which GC exhibits both stimulatory and inhibitory effects on it [45]. GC can modulate the expression of the LH receptor (LHR) on the gonads, and it also can inhibit the synthesis of testosterone (T), estrogen (E2), and progesterone (P). Hence, it can easily dysregulate these signals and cause profound fertility problems in both ovarian function during ovulation and uterine function during fertilization, implantation, and pregnancy [43].

3.3.2 Via the peripheral tissue

In addition to the effects of GC and GR on the central nervous system, GR expression also has been demonstrated in the peripheral tissue [35]. Mifepristone, a potent high-affinity GR antagonist, also implied the effects of GC regulating embryo attachment and invasion [46]. However, direct evidence implicating GR signaling in uterine biology has been described only recently. The study suggested that decreased blastocyst implantation rate and subsequent defects in stromal cell decidualization were found out in a uterine-specific glucocorticoid receptor (GR) knockout (uterine GR KO) mouse. As a master regulator, GC repressed some important gene expression and eventually influenced the uterine environment [35].

4. Hypothalamus-pituitary-thyroid axis

There are three dominant hormones within the hypothalamus-pituitary-thyroid axis (HPT axis), such as thyrotropin-releasing hormone (TRH), thyrotropin-stimulating hormone (TSH), and thyroid hormone (TH: T3 and T4) [3]. When it comes to pregnancy accompanied with thyroid disease, we always ascribe subfertility and recurrent miscarriage to either hypothyroidism or hyperthyroidism [47]. In in vivo studies, it has been demonstrated that hypothyroidism might have a dual effect on pregnancy, by influencing implantation at a very early stage and regulating placental development at the later stage [48]. Moreover, thyroid hormone receptors, expressed in the endometrium and trophoblast during implantation, can influence the feto-maternal interface [49]. In in vitro studies, it has been proven that TH is involved in the bidirectional cross talk between the blastocyst and endometrium during implantation. In hypothyroid females, lower levels of both ISP1 and ISP2 (two key regulators of embryo implantation) could be found in the uterus [48]. Furthermore, TH impacts both the endometrium and the trophoblast, via either directly or indirectly through TH effects on the synthesis and activity of implantation-mediating molecules [50]. Although a research indicated that when TSH value was below 2.5 mIU/L, no association varying TSH values and implantation was detected [51]. TH receptors (TRs) and TSH receptors (TSHRs) were broadly presented in the feto-maternal unit [50] and even increase the expression of TSHR, TRa1, TRa2, and TRb1 in endometrial cells during peri-implantation [52]. Moreover, TH synthesis is related to several transcripts, including prolyl 4-hydroxylase beta (P4HB), a molecular chaperone involved in endocytosis of immature thyroglobulin (Tg) molecules, thyroid peroxidase (TPO), and Tg, which also could be discovered in the endometrium [53].

Beyond that, hypothyroidism can result in development of reduced endometrial thickness, because of reducing the uterine cells' estrogenic response [54]. In addition to affecting the proliferation and maturation of endometrial tissue, TH also could have profound effects on the regulation of the HPG axis and subsequently on implantation [55]. Angiogenesis and endometrium remodeling are considered as pivotal events for successful implantation, decidualization, and placentation, while it has been demonstrated that TH can exert an important role in angiogenesis via both genomic and non-genomic mechanisms in a variety of animal models [56]. Besides, TH regulates integrin $\alpha\nu\beta3$, a class of cell adhesion molecules (CAMs) that interacts with extracellular matrix (ECM) ligands, matrix metalloproteinases (MMPs), and other CAMs, playing a critical role in the cascade of events to successful implantation [57].

In summary, it is clearly suggested that both TSH and TH are essential players in the mechanism of regulating implantation based on current experimental and clinical evidences. However, less evidence shows the influence of TRH on the implantation procedure; thus further exploration needs to be continued.

5. Hypothalamo-neurohypophyseal system

Hormones from the posterior lobe of the pituitary also play an essential role in neuroendocrine and implantation. The hypothalamo-neurohypophyseal system is composed of the hypothalamus and posterior pituitary, regarded as the site for secretion of neurohypophysial hormones, classically including oxytocin and vasopressin [58].

It is well established that apt uterine contractile activity uterus is vital to successful implantation, and it has been proven that both oxytocin and vasopressin receptors are expressed in the uterus, which are closely relevant to the contractile activity of the uterus [49]. Both oxytocin and vasopressin receptors belong to the class I family of G-coupled receptors, regulating uterus contraction via a central or peripheral pathway [59]. So far, massive research literature indicated that oxytocin and vasopressin antagonist treatment was effective in priming of the uterus for implantation and consequently improved the implantation rate after IVF [58, 60–62].

Atosiban, a mixed vasopressin V1a and oxytocin receptor antagonist, have been demonstrated to improve uterine receptivity, provide a decrease in uterine contractile activity, and increase endometrial blood perfusion in women undergoing embryo transfer [58]. Another important effect of atosiban is to decrease endometrial perfusion and embryonic survival rate by inhibiting the stimulation of the endometrial production of prostaglandin F2a in an animal model [63]. With the beneficial of improving uterine environment, atosiban can be a specific treatment for the improvement of implantation rate following IVF-ET [64]. Thereby, the novel class of drugs based on these two receptors and its relative pathway for improving implantation rate and pregnancy outcomes still need to be further explored.

6. Neuroendocrine systems improve implantation rate in IVF-ET

Infertility gradually becomes an epidemic problem and brings an enormous burden on about 10% of the couples in child-bearing age [65]. Implantation concerns frequently arise in couples with infertility, especially in the setting of assisted reproductive technology (ART) cycles [4]. Regardless of the impressive development in ART, there are still approximately 10–15% of the infertile couples suffering from recurrent implantation failure (RIF) [2].

According to the literature, factors involved in recurrent implantation failure can be summarized in three aspects such as decreased endometrial receptivity, defective embryonic developments, and others [2, 4]. However, only the evidence about different axes of hormones from neuroendocrine influencing the procedure of implantation has been concluded in this paper, and it mainly focuses on the aspect of decreasing maternal endometrium receptivity but less on blastocyst (**Table 1**).

Furthermore, the relevant literatures of ACTH, TRH, as well as TSH on implantation procedure are less, and their mechanisms are not elaborated enough. Hence, studies aiming to better define the association between neuroendocrine system and implantation processes should be further investigated, which may lead to further therapeutic intervention, thereby optimizing embryo implantation and eventually improving the success rate following IVF-ET.

HPG axis	GnRH and GnRH-II	Altered expression of adhesive molecules
	LH and FSH	-
	Estrogen and Progesterone	Endometrium thickness
		Altered expression of adhesive molecules
		Immunological factors
		Prevent thrombus formation
HPA axis	CRH	Modulating HPG axis
		Altered expression of adhesive molecules
		Immunological factors
	ACTH	Modulating HPG axis
	GCs	Modulating HPG axis
		Regulating uterine environment
		Embryo attachment and invasion
HPT axis	TRH	-
	TSH	Feto-maternal interface
	TH	Feto-maternal interface
		Endometrium thickness
		Modulating HPG axis
		Angiogenesis
		Altered expression of adhesive molecules
Hypothalamus-neurohypophyseal system	Oxytocin &Vasopressin	Uterine contractile activity
		Endometrium perfusion

Table 1.
Mainly aspects of neuroendocrine hormones involved in improving the condition of RIF.

Author details

Fenting Liu and Rong Li*
Center for Reproductive Medicine, Department of Obstetrics and Gynecology, Peking University Third Hospital, Beijing, China

*Address all correspondence to: roseli001@sina.com

References

[1] León-Olea M et al. Current concepts in neuroendocrine disruption. General and Comparative Endocrinology. 2014;**203**:158-173

[2] Margalioth EJ et al. Investigation and treatment of repeated implantation failure following IVF-ET. Human Reproduction. 2006;**21**(12):3036-3043

[3] Musumeci G, Castorina S, Castrogiovanni P, Loreto C, Leonardi R, Aiello FC, et al. A journey through the pituitary gland: Development, structure and function, with emphasis on embryo-foetal and later development. Acta Histochemica. 2015;**117**(4-5):355-366

[4] Simon A, Laufer N. Repeated implantation failure: Clinical approach. Fertility and Sterility. 2012;**97**(5):1039-1043

[5] Maggi R et al. GnRH and GnRH receptors in the pathophysiology of the human female reproductive system. Human Reproduction Update. 2016;**22**(3):358-381

[6] Wu HM et al. Gonadotropin-releasing hormone type II (GnRH-II) agonist regulates the motility of human decidual endometrial stromal cells: Possible effect on embryo implantation and pregnancy. Biology of Reproduction. 2015;**92**(4):98

[7] Yu B et al. The role of peripheral gonadotropin-releasing hormone receptors in female reproduction. Fertility and Sterility. 2011;**95**(2):465-473

[8] Barbieri RL. The endocrinology of the menstrual cycle. In: Rosenwaks Z, Wassarman P, editors. Human Fertility. Methods in Molecular Biology (Methods and Protocols). Vol. 1154. New York, NY: Humana Press; 2014. pp. 145-169

[9] Millar RP et al. A novel mammalian receptor for the evolutionarily conserved type II gonadotropin-releasing hormone. Proceedings of the National Academy of Sciences of the United States of America. 2001;**98**:9636-9641

[10] Millar RP. GnRH-II and type-II GnRH receptors. Trends in Endocrinology and Metabolism. 2003;**14**:35-43

[11] Meng Y et al. Effects of GnRH antagonist on endometrial protein profiles in the window of implantation. Proteomics. 2014;**14**(20):2350-2235

[12] Thor H, Matheus R, Esteves SC, Peter H. GnRH agonist trigger and LH activity luteal phase support versus hCG trigger and conventional luteal phase support in fresh embryo transfer IVF/ICSI cycles—A systematic PRISMA review and meta-analysis. Frontiers in Endocrinology. 2017;**8**:116

[13] Lessey BA, Young SL. Homeostasis imbalance in the endometrium of women with implantation defects: The role of estrogen and progesterone. Seminars in Reproductive Medicine. 2014;**32**(5):365-375

[14] Ghosh D, De P, Sengupta J. Luteal phase ovarian oestrogen is not essential for implantation and maintenance of pregnancy from surrogate embryo transfer in the rhesus monkey. Human Reproduction. 1994;**9**:629

[15] Donaghay M, Lessey BA. Uterine receptivity: Alterations associated with benign gynecological disease. Seminars in Reproduction Medicine. 2007;**25**(6):461-475

[16] Groll JM, Usadi RS, Lessey BA, Lininger R, Young SL, Fritz MA. Effects of variations in serum

estradiol concentrations on secretory endometrial development and function in experimentally induced cycles in normal women. Fertility and Sterility. 2009;**92**(6):2058-2061

[17] Young SL. Oestrogen and progesterone action on endometrium: A translational approach to understanding endometrial receptivity. Reproductive Biomedicine Online. 2013;**27**(5):497-505

[18] Liang XH et al. Egr1 protein acts downstream of estrogen-leukemia inhibitory factor (LIF)-STAT3 pathway and plays a role during implantation through targeting Wnt4. Journal of Biological Chemistry. 2014;**289**(34):23534-23545

[19] Yoshinaga K. Progesterone and its downstream molecules as blastocyst implantation essential factors. American Journal of Reproductive Immunology. 2014;**72**(2):117-128

[20] Kobayashi R et al. The window of implantation is closed by estrogen via insulin-like growth factor 1 pathway. Journal of Reproduction & Infertility. 2017;**18**(2):231-241

[21] Liu X, Nie J, Guo SW. Elevated immunoreactivity to tissue factor and its association with dysmenorrhea severity and the amount of menses in adenomyosis. Human Reproduction. 2011;**26**:337-345

[22] Nordengren J, Pilka R, Noskova V, et al. Differential localization and expression of urokinase plasminogen activator (uPA), its receptor (uPAR) and its inhibitor PAI-1 mRNA and protein in endometrial tissue during the menstrual cycle. Molecular Human Reproduction. 2004;**10**:655-663

[23] van der Linden M, Buckingham K, Farquhar C, Kremer JA, Metwally M. Luteal phase support for assisted reproduction cycles. The Cochrane Database of Systematic Reviews. 2015;7:CD009154

[24] Tan O, Bukulmez O. Biochemistry, molecular biology and cell biology of gonadotropin-releasing hormone antagonists. Current Opinion of Obstetrics and Gynecology. 2011;**23**:238-244

[25] Huang F, Wang H, Zou Y, Liu Q, Cao J, Yin T. Effect of GnRH-II on the ESC proliferation, apoptosis and VEGF secretion in patients with endometriosis in vitro. International Journal of Clinical and Experimental Pathology. 2013;**6**(11):2487-2496

[26] Naruse K, Lash GB, Otun H, et al. Localization of matrix metalloproteinase (MMP)-2, MMP-9 and tissue inhibitors for MMPs (TIMPs) in uterine natural killer cells in early human pregnancy. Human Reproduction. 2009;**24**(3):553-561

[27] Hillhouse EW, Grammatopoulos DK. The molecular mechanisms underlying the regulation of the biological activity of corticotropin-releasing hormone receptors: Implications for physiology and pathophysiology. Endocrine Reviews. 2006;**27**:260-286

[28] Vergetaki A, Jeschke U, Vrekoussis T, Taliouri E, Sabatini L, Papakonstanti EA, et al. Galectin-1 overexpression in endometriosis and its regulation by neuropeptides (CRH, UCN) indicating its important role in reproduction and inflammation. PLoS ONE. 2014;**9**(12):e114229

[29] Phumsatitpong C, Moenter SM. Estradiol-dependent stimulation and suppression of gonadotropin-releasing hormone neuron firing activity by corticotropin-releasing hormone in female mice. Endocrinology. 2018;**159**(1):414-425

[30] Kalantaridou SN et al. Corticotropin-releasing hormone, stress and human reproduction: An update. Journal of Reproduction Immunology. 2010;**85**(1):33-39

[31] Makrigiannakis A, Zoumakis E, Kalantaridou S, Coutifaris C, Margioris AN, Coukos G, et al. Corticotropin-releasing hormone promotes blastocyst implantation and early maternal tolerance. Nature Immunology. 2011;**2**:1018-1024

[32] Bamberger AM, Minas V, Kalantaridou SN, Radde J, Sadeghian H, Loning T, et al. Corticotropin-releasing hormone modulates human trophoblast invasion through carcinoembryonic antigen-related cell adhesion molecule-1 regulation. American Journal of Pathology. 2006;**168**:141-150

[33] Brann DW, Mahesh VB. Role of corticosteroids in female reproduction. FASEB Journal. 1991;**5**(12):2691-2698

[34] Chatterjee A, Harper MJ. Interruption of implantation and gestation in rats by reserpine, chlorpromazine and ACTH: Possible mode of action. Endocrinology. 1970;**5**(87):966-969

[35] Whirledge SD et al. Uterine glucocorticoid receptors are critical for fertility in mice through control of embryo implantation and decidualization. Proceedings of the National Academy of Sciences. 2015;**112**(49):15166-15171

[36] Boomsma CM, Keay SD, Macklon NS. Peri-implantation glucocorticoid administration for assisted reproductive technology cycles. Cochrane Database of Systematic Reviews. 2007;**24**(1):CD005996

[37] Duong HT, Piotrowska-Tomala KK, Acosta TJ, Bah MM, Sinderewicz E, Majewska M, et al. Effects of cortisol on pregnancy rate and corpus luteum function in heifers: An in vivo study. Journal of Reproduction and Development. 2012;**58**(2):223-230

[38] Geraghty AC, Kaufer D. Glucocorticoid regulation of reproduction. In: Wang JC, Harris C, editors. Glucocorticoid Signaling. Advances in Experimental Medicine and Biology. Vol. 872. New York, NY: Springer; 2015. pp. 253-278

[39] Mohsen A et al. A novel non-genomic glucocorticoid signaling mediated by a membrane palmitoylated glucocorticoid receptor cross talks with GnRH in gonadotrope cells. Scientific Reports. 2017;**1**(7):1537

[40] Gore AC et al. Glucocorticoid repression of the reproductive axis: Effects on GnRH and gonadotropin subunit mRNA levels. Molecular and Cellular Endocrinology. 2006;**256**(1-2):40-48

[41] Ciechanowska M, Łapot M, Paruszewska E, et al. The influence of dopaminergic system inhibition on biosynthesis of gonadotrophin-releasing hormone (GnRH) and GnRH receptor in anoestrous sheep; hierarchical role of kisspeptin and RFamide-related peptide-3 (RFRP-3). Reproduction, Fertility and Development. 2018;**30**(4):672-680

[42] Takumi K, Iijima N, Higo S, Ozawa H. Immunohistochemical analysis of the colocalization of corticotropin-releasing hormone receptor and glucocorticoid receptor in kisspeptin neurons in the hypothalamus of female rats. Neuroscience Letters. 2012;**531**(1):40-45

[43] Whirledge S, Cidlowski JA. A role for glucocorticoids in stress-impaired reproduction: Beyond the hypothalamus and pituitary. Endocrinology. 2013;**154**(12):4450-4468

[44] Du Ruisseau P, Taché Y, Brazeau P, Collu R. Effects of chronic

immobilization stress on pituitary hormone secretion, on hypothalamic factor levels, and on pituitary responsiveness to LHRH and TRH in female rats. Neuroendocrinology. 1979;**29**(2):90-99

[45] Michael AE, Pester LA, Curtis P, Shaw RW, Edwards CR, Cooke BA. Direct inhibition of ovarian steroidogenesis by cortisol and the modulatory role of 11 beta-hydroxysteroid dehydrogenase. Clinical Endocrinology. 1993;**38**(6):641-644

[46] Couzinet B, Le Strat N, Ulmann A, Baulieu EE, Schaison G. Termination of early pregnancy by the progesterone antagonist RU 486 (Mifepristone). New England Journal of Medicine. 1986;**315**(25):1565-1570

[47] Twig G, Shina A, Amital H, Shoenfeld Y. Pathogenesis of infertility and recurrent pregnancy loss in thyroid autoimmunity. Journal of Autoimmunity. 2012;**38**(2-3):J275-JJ28

[48] Piccirilli D, Baldini E, Massimiani M, Camaioni A, Salustri A, Bernardini R, et al. Thyroid hormone regulates protease expression and activation of notch signaling in implantation and embryo development. Journal of Endocrinology. 2018;**236**(1):1

[49] van den Boogaard E, Vissenberg RLand JA, van Wely M, van der Post JA, Goddijn M, Bisschop PH. Significance of (sub)clinical thyroid dysfunction and thyroid autoimmunity before conception and in early pregnancy: A systematic review. Human Reproduction Update. 2011;**17**(5):605-619

[50] Colicchia M et al. Molecular basis of thyrotropin and thyroid hormone action during implantation and early development. Human Reproduction Update. 2014;**20**(6):884-904

[51] Green KA et al. Investigating the optimal preconception TSH range for patients undergoing IVF when controlling for embryo quality. Journal of Assisted Reproduction and Genetics. 2015;**32**(10):1469-1476

[52] Sayem ASM et al. Effects of thyroxine on expression of proteins related to thyroid hormone functions (TR-α, TR-β, RXR and ERK1/2) in uterus during peri-implantation period. Biomedicine & Pharmacotherapy. 2017;**96**:1016-1021

[53] Catalano RD, Critchley HO, Heikinheimo O, Baird DT, Hapangama D, Sherwin JRA, et al. Mifepristone induced progesterone withdrawal reveals novel regulatory pathways in human endometrium. Molecular Human Reproduction. 2007;**13**:641-654

[54] Inuwa I, Williams MA. Morphometric study on the uterine horn and thyroid gland in hypothyroid and thyroxin treated hypothyroid rats. Journal of Anatomy. 1996;**188**:383-393

[55] Redmond GP. Thyroid dysfunction and women's reproductive health. Thyroid. 2004;**14**:S5-S15

[56] Yalcin M, Dyskin E, Lansing L, Bharali DJ, Mousa SS, Bridoux A, et al. Tetraiodothyroacetic acid (tetrac) and nanoparticulate tetrac arrest growth of medullary carcinoma of the thyroid. Journal of Clinical Endocrinology and Metabolism. 2010;**95**:1972-1980

[57] Tei C, Maruyama T, Kuji N, Miyazaki T, Mikami M, Yoshimura Y. Reduced expression of alphavbeta3 integrin in the endometrium of unexplained infertility patients with recurrent IVF-ET failures: Improvement by danazol treatment. Journal of Assisted Reproduction and Genetics. 2003;**20**:13-20

[58] Pierzynski P. Oxytocin and vasopressin V(1A) receptors as new therapeutic targets in assisted

reproduction. Reproductive Biomedicine Online. 2011;**22**(1):9-16

[59] Chini B, Fanelli F. Molecular basis of ligand binding and receptor activation in the oxytocin and vasopressin receptor family. Experimental Physiology. 2010;**85, s1**:59s-66s

[60] Chou PY et al. Use of an oxytocin antagonist in in vitro fertilization-embryo transfer for women with repeated implantation failure: A retrospective study. Taiwanese Journal of Obstetrics & Gynecology. 2011;**50**(2):136-140

[61] Khairy M et al. The effect of peri-implantation administration of uterine relaxing agents in assisted reproduction treatment cycles: A systematic review and meta-analysis. Reproductive Biomedicine Online. 2016;**32**(4):362-376

[62] Kim SK et al. Efficacy of oxytocin antagonist infusion in improving in vitro fertilization outcomes on the day of embryo transfer: A meta-analysis. Clinical and Experimental Reproductive Medicine. 2016;**43**(4):233-239

[63] Lemaster JW, Seals RC, Hopkins FM, Schrick FN. Effects of administration of oxytocin on embryonic survival in progestogen supplemented cattle. Prostaglandins and Other Lipid Mediators. 1999;**57**:259-268

[64] Moraloglu O et al. Treatment with oxytocin antagonists before embryo transfer may increase implantation rates after IVF. Reproductive Biomedicine Online. 2010;**21**(3):338-343

[65] Boivin J, Bunting L, Collins JA, Nygren KG. International estimates of infertility prevalence and treatment-seeking: Potential need and demand for infertility medical care. Human Reproduction. 2007;**22**:1506-1512

Section 4

Embryo Cryopreservation and ART Outcome

Chapter 8

The Present and Future of Embryo Cryopreservation

Iavor K. Vladimirov, Desislava Tacheva and Vladislav Dobrinov

Abstract

Embryo freezing technologies have widely been used in human IVF practice and in animal industry. In this chapter, we will review the development of embryo freezing technology and the application of the method, which will concentrate on discussion of the arguments in favor of and against freezing, as well as the latest results of success rates, comparing them with the other basic assisted reproductive technologies methods. Then, we will present our viewpoint for the future application of embryo freezing methods and their place in reproductive medicine. The analysis of facts and suggestions should enable researchers to rethink the position of cryobiology in reproductive medicine. It should be considered that the method of cryopreservation is not only a technology for storing embryos but also a method of embryo treatment that can potentially improve the success rates in infertile couples. There is also a theory that describes the "treatment" effect of freezing an embryo, which may explain the higher success rates of frozen embryo transfer (FET) compared to fresh embryo transfer (ET). The authors of the "Theory about the Embryo-Cryo treatment" believe that freezing and thawing could activate endogenous survival and repair mechanisms in preimplantation embryos.

Keywords: embryo, cryobiology, embryo treatment, frozen embryo transfer, ART methods

1. Introduction

During the last couple of decades, assisted reproductive technologies (ART) have become one of the fastest developing branches of medicine. Since they are the main method of fertility treatment, much research has been done in this area. Enormous amount of work has been done to elucidate the benefits of cryopreservation of stem cells, embryos, gametes, tissues, and organs. The idea of maintaining the viability of living reproductive cells and tissues of various species after long-term storage provides a chance for animal and human reproductive applications [1, 2]. Due to the constantly improving cryopreservation techniques, we are now able to preserve cells and tissues by cooling them to extremely low temperatures, such as −195.79°C (the boiling point of the liquid nitrogen). Cooling down biological objects to such degrees prevents any biological activity, including all the biochemical reactions involved in cell death.

Among the biggest scientific achievements, cryopreservation of embryos came into prominence more than 45 years ago [3, 4]. In 1972, Whittingham and associates

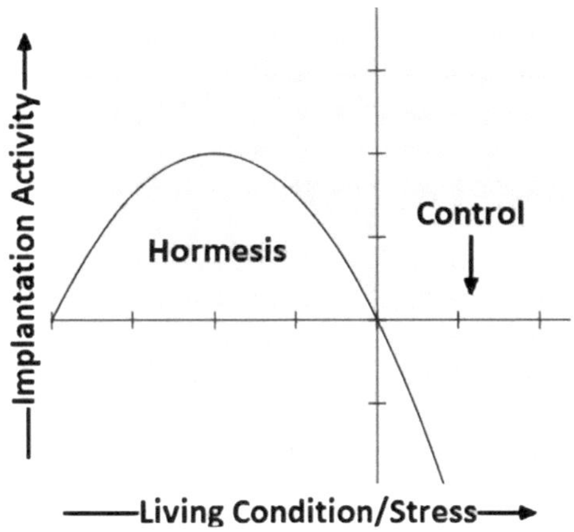

Figure 1.
Mechanism of hormesis (License: 4371720640523).

and Wilmut succeeded in cryopreservation of eight-cell mouse embryos [3, 4]. Since that time, vast number of embryos from various mammalian species have been frozen, thawed, and eventually transferred successfully, thus proving the benefits from this ART procedure. In 1983, Trounson and Mohr achieved the first human pregnancy from frozen embryo with the same procedure used successfully for cryopreservation of mouse and cow embryos [5].

Without doubt, the successful cryopreservation of embryos has greatly improved the chances for a successful outcome after a single cycle of ovarian stimulation and in vitro fertilization (IVF). There is also a theory that describes the "treatment" effect of freezing an embryo, which may explain the higher success rates of frozen embryo transfer (FET) compared to fresh embryo transfer (ET). The authors of the "Theory about the Embryo-Cryo treatment" believe that freezing and thawing could activate endogenous survival and repair mechanisms in pre-implantation embryos [6]. The idea is that the thawing process induces low levels of stress, which leads to hormesis. This controlled stress could lead to the repair of mitochondrial damage and protein misfolding. This theory may explain the higher success rate of FET compared to fresh ET in women of advanced reproductive age, the higher miscarriage rate after thawed blastocyst transfers compared to thawed early cleavage embryos transfers and the higher perinatal parameters of children born after FET (**Figure 1**).

While much has been discovered about embryo cryopreservation, there are still many things that have to be defined more accurately, such as the freezing medium composition or the stage of the embryo during freezing. Embryo freezing methods are constantly being improved, but they, as well as the freezing equipment, require improvements. Scientists are looking for answers to these and many more questions while the final goal remains clear—successful cryopreservation followed by as high as possible pregnancy rates. In this chapter, we will try to present the most important aspects of cryopreservation. In the end, we hope that the potential of cryobiology in reproductive medicine will have been acknowledged.

2. Cryobiology and reproductive medicine

Cryobiology represents a branch of biology which studies the effects of low temperatures on organisms, biological systems, or biological materials. Those low temperatures range from hypothermic to cryogenic (−150°C or lower).

While cryobiology is mainly focused on the “living world,” in the last decades, it has been expanded to involve treatment of nonliving things, as well. With the development of highly sophisticated cryobiological techniques, like cryosurgery, embryo and gamete preservation and others, this biological branch has the potential to affect everyone's lives in the future.

The idea of freezing human gametes for their future use encouraged scientists to incorporate cryobiology in the field of reproductive medicine. Polge et al. in 1949 have been recognized as the first researchers who cryopreserved spermatozoa while using glycerol as a cryoprotectant [7], although Bernstein and Petropavlovski 12 years earlier demonstrated that glycerol has a cryoprotective role in the cryopreservation of spermatozoa [8]. Encouraged by those findings and driven by the potential benefits of freezing human gametes and embryos, scientists soon began to study much more in the biology of cryopreservation. Rapid progress was made, and the first birth from the use of human frozen spermatozoa was achieved in 1954 [9]. In those days, scientists used spermatozoa for their cryopreservation studies, since they have motility, which was useful when assessing the vitality of the frozen/thawed probe. Nowadays, cryopreservation of spermatozoa could be achieved easily and is a routine procedure, performed worldwide.

Freezing oocytes was much harder to achieve, and it took scientists some time. Chen in 1986 reported the first pregnancy, resulting from slow freezing and rapid thawing of human oocytes using DMSO (dimethyl sulfoxide) as a cryoprotectant [10]. However, earlier concerns were raised regarding damage to the meiotic spindle, loss of cortical granules, and the low success rates as compared to the relative success of embryo cryopreservation, which led to little interest in oocyte freezing until 1990s [11]. During those times, Bernard et al. and other researchers demonstrated that reasonable oocyte thaw survival [12] and subsequent fertilization could be achieved [13]. Gradually, interest was raising, and through hard work, oocyte freezing is now also a routine procedure.

One of the very important attainments that cryobiology has achieved is the ability to successfully freeze and thaw human embryos. Scientists first discovered how to successfully freeze an embryo, and only after that, they achieved successful oocyte cryopreservation. Whittingham et al. achieved the first successful embryo cryopreservation when the research group froze mouse embryos in polyvinylpyrrolidone (PVP) [3]. The first baby born after a frozen/thawed blastocyst transfer was reported by Cohen et al. in 1985 [14]. Embryo cryopreservation is now a routine procedure and there is sufficient published data supporting its effectiveness.

3. Embryo cryopreservation

Cryopreservation of embryos is a very delicate procedure, which also hides some risks to the things that are frozen. During the freezing process, embryos are exposed to physical stress, caused either by the direct effects of the low temperature or by physical changes induced by ice formation.

The direct effects of the low temperature may induce damage to cell structure and function. The mitotic spindle is especially sensitive to cold shock injuries. The extent of the damage, caused by the freezing procedure, depends on various factors, like the shape and size of the cells, the membrane composition, and its permeability. All these factors are variable and are species specific. Embryos and oocytes have the ability to repair some damage in order to survive and develop properly.

The formation of ice crystals is detrimental to cells. The damage that the cells suffer is not due to the crystallization of ice but rather due to the high concentration of solutes occurring when water is removed in order to form ice [15].

Cryoprotectants (CPAs) act to reduce cellular damage by increasing the volume of the unfrozen residual phase. When the first cryopreservation experiments took place, two opposing methods had been developed simultaneously—a method of slow freezing of the cells and vitrification. Since these methods were very different, scientists started to compare them, in order to elucidate their benefits and drawbacks. Vitrification offers the possibility of eliminating the formation of ice crystals [16], and over the years, it has gradually replaced slow freezing as the preferred method of cryopreservation in the field of reproductive medicine. The main reason behind this fact is that vitrification achieves better survival rates, and moreover, it is less time consuming to perform and does not require highly specialized and expensive equipment like in the slow freezing technique.

3.1 Cryoprotectants

Cryoprotectants (CPAs) are substances that protect cells/tissues from the damage that may occur during the freezing process. In order to achieve successful cryopreservation of any biological material, the freezing protocols must be optimized, starting with the correct choice of CPA and ending with the thawing process and post-thawing handling of the material. The choice of the most appropriate CPA for a certain freezing procedure is difficult to make, because it must take into consideration the CPA's toxicity, permeability, and also its physicochemical properties. CPAs are widely used to improve the cryosurvival rates, although their mechanism of action is not fully understood. One of their properties is to lower the freezing point of a certain solution, while also protecting the cell membrane during the freezing process. CPAs may also act to stabilize intracellular protein structure. As mentioned earlier, freezing an embryo is a very delicate procedure and embryos may be damaged by chilling, fracturing, ice formation (intra and extracellular), the chemical toxicity of CPAs, osmotic swelling, and osmotic shrinkage [17]. Chilling injuries can lead to changes in lipid-rich membranes and can also result in cytoskeletal disorganization. The mechanical effect of a solidified solution may cause fracture damage, especially to embryos. One of the first documented studies that introduced the concept of cryoprotectants was that of Polge et al. [7, 18], which assessed the use of glycerol in sperm freezing, and it also provided the basis of many future investigations concerning CPAs.

Regarding their structure, CPAs are small molecular weight solutes possessing high aqueous solubility and polar groups that interact weakly with water [19]. CPAs are generally divided into two groups based on their ability to penetrate through the cell membrane—permeating (PM) and nonpermeating (NPM). It is important to point out that PM and NPM cryoprotectants are often used together in order to achieve a successful cryopreservation of cells and tissues. In fact, the core of a cryopreservation solution is made of a mixture of those CPAs, and it also includes various components, like some salts, pH buffers, and others. In the PM group are included some of the most studied CPAs like glycerol (G), ethylene glycol (EG), dimethyl sulfoxide (DMSO), formamide, propylene glycol (PG), and others. PM cryoprotectants are the most important component in the vitrification solution. G and EG are the most commonly used PM CPAs. NPM cryoprotectants include saccharides, polyvinylpyrrolidone (PVP), polyethylene glycol (PEG), and others. They are large molecules, usually polymers. Sucrose is the most commonly used NPM cryoprotectant. The effect of these NPM agents is the dehydration of the cells by osmosis. They also act to stabilize the cell's membrane [20] and aid the entry of PM cryoprotectants [21]. Moreover, NPM CPAs are added during the thawing process as they act to reduce the osmotic shock.

Nowadays, there are many freezing media produced by biotechnology companies, which are made by mixing various substances to achieve maximum cryoprotection. The composition of these freezing media varies greatly, since there is no "perfect formula" and therefore the search goes on.

3.2 Methods

Practically, two methods for embryo cryopreservation have been used—slow freezing and vitrification. Here, we will briefly review both of them and we will discuss their positives and negatives.

3.2.1 Slow freezing

Slow freezing is a conventional cryopreservation method, which is based on a slow cooling rate and use of a low concentration of CPAs. This leads to less toxicity to cells/tissues; however, it does not eliminate ice formation. In 1972, two scientific groups published the first survival of murine embryos after slow freezing [3, 4] and live offspring [3]. Nowadays, after the introduction of the vitrification method, slow freezing is gradually being replaced.

Protocols based on the slow freezing method include an equilibrating step, during which the cells or tissues are placed in an aqueous solution containing PM CPAs in low concentrations (1.0–1.5 M) and sucrose (0.1 M) before which they are placed in ampules or straws. After the exposure to CPAs, initial cellular dehydration is observed followed by a return to isotonic volume with the permeation of CPA and water. After loading the specimen in the straw/ampulla, the temperature is being lowered down slowly with the aid of a controlled rate freezing machine which allows samples to be cooled at different rates, and finally, the frozen objects are placed in liquid nitrogen for storage. The slow cooling is performed to ensure that the cells/tissues are dehydrated before intracellular ice formation occurs. However, the optimal rate of cooling varies greatly among cells and tissue types [22]. A crucial step during the slow freezing protocol is the so-called ice crystal seeding which can be performed either manually or automatically. It takes place after the ampules/straws, preloaded with the embryos, are cooled below the melting point of the solution which is around −5 to −7°C. At these temperatures, solutions remain unfrozen due to the supercooling (lowering the temperature of a solution below its freezing point without extracellular ice formation). Supercooling leads to improper cell dehydration and to avoid such fate, most commonly manual ice nucleation is performed by touching the ampules/straws with a prechilled with liquid nitrogen cold object like forceps which leads to ice crystal formation. In this way, the remaining water in the cells is driven away due to the osmotic imbalance, caused by the formation of ice crystals. After ice crystal seeding, the process of slow freezing continues at various cooling rates. When the temperature has reached values ranging from −30 to −80°C depending on the protocol, the ampules/straws are plunged into liquid nitrogen.

In conclusion, we must say that despite the acceptable results achieved by slow freezing, it also has its negatives, for example, it is time consuming, as freezing an embryo usually takes between 2 and 3 hours depending on the cooling rate. Furthermore, it requires expensive controlled-rate freezers.

3.2.2 Vitrification

Vitrification is an alternative approach to the slow freezing method for the cryopreservation of embryos/gametes. Vitrification differs from slow freezing in that it avoids the formation of ice crystals both intracellularly and extracellularly [23]. This method is easier to conduct, does not require expensive equipment like programmable freezers, and is not that time consuming when compared to the conventional slow freezing.

Physically speaking, vitrification is the solidification of a solution at low temperatures by elevation in viscosity during cooling and not by ice crystallization [24, 25]. The first successful vitrification of embryos was published in 1985 by Rall and Fahy, who froze mouse embryos using DMSO, PEG, and acetamide [23]. Commonly used freezing solutions for vitrifications are composed of permeating CPA (EG, DMSO, G, acetamide, PG, with a concentration of over 4 M) and nonpermeating CPA (most commonly sucrose, >0.5 M). After numerous experiments and further improvements of the vitrification technique, like replacement of DMSO with EG and mixture of several CPAs [26], vitrification was applied to human embryos and live births were achieved with both blastocyst and cleavage stage embryos [27, 28]. Assisted hatching (AH) was added to the freezing/thawing procedure and is performed before the transfer of vitrified embryos. It was reported that AH is beneficial in vitrification cycles by increasing pregnancy and implantation rates [29]. Although several methods of AH had been developed—mechanical, piezo, chemical, and laser, the latter turns out to be the most used one with one of its main advantages lies in minimizing the exposure of embryos outside the incubator. A recent meta-analysis conducted in 2016 encompassing 36 randomized controlled trials and 6459 participants reported increased clinical pregnancy rate and multiple pregnancy rate in couples after AH and nonsignificant difference in miscarriage rates between the AH group and the control one [30]. Despite fears about the safety of AH and the increased chance of multiple pregnancies, many IVF facilities apply the procedure on every thawed embryo. The idea behind this is to improve the implantation and clinical pregnancy rates especially in women with history of repeated IVF failure. Embryos with thicker zona pellucida could benefit the most after AH. A large study by Knudtson et al. with more than 150,000 FET cycles reported a slightly decreased live birth rate in the first autologous FET cycle after AH [31]. Therefore, the application of AH should be carefully considered, and prospective studies should be carried out in order to elucidate its benefits and negatives.

The vitrification protocols for embryo freezing consist of several steps. In the first place, embryos are exposed to high concentrations of CPAs, after that, they are loaded into carriers, most commonly straws, and finally those straws are cooled as fast as possible, reaching a cooling rate of thousands of degrees per minute. To achieve vitrification of solutions, there must be an increase in both the cooling rates and the concentration of CPAs. Those two factors are inverse proportionally connected since, the higher the cooling rate, the lower the required CPA. It is important to mention that there are some concerns regarding the use of high concentrations of CPAs, because they could harm the cells during vitrification. That is why a mixture of CPAs is used during vitrification in order to reduce this toxicity.

Vitrification techniques include the so-called "open" and "closed" systems or carriers. The idea behind them is unambiguous, and with the open carriers, the embryos are directly exposed to the liquid nitrogen, which increases the cooling rate, but hides a potential risk of cross contamination of the probe during the storage in liquid nitrogen. On the other hand, the closed systems isolate the sample from the liquid nitrogen which lowers substantially the risk of contamination; however, the cooling rate is inferior compared to the open carriers. There are dozens of different carrier devices available commercially, but there are not many comprehensive studies that compare the carriers and their efficiency. When comparing open and closed systems (VitriSafe carrier, open and closed variation) for blastocyst freezing, a prospective study by Panagiotidis et al. documented no significant difference between the two carrier systems [32], which highlights the importance of the thawing process. Kuwayama et al. compared open (Cryotop) and closed

(CryoTip) systems for the vitrification of blastocysts and also found no significant difference (survival rate 97 and 93% for Cryotop and CryoTip, respectively, deliveries 51 and 48%). These observations support the thesis that closed systems are comparable to open ones, because they also reduce the risk of cross contamination.

We hope that vitrification will be optimized in the near future and questions regarding the composition of the vitrification solution, the most appropriate carrier type, and others would be answered in due time.

3.2.3 Method comparison

In the pool of studies that compare slow freezing of embryos and vitrification, Kuwayama et al. reported that vitrification of 5881 human PN stage embryos resulted in 100% survival, 93% cleavage, and 52% blastocyst rates. In contrast, after slow freezing of 1944 PN stage embryos, the results were 89% survival, 90% cleavage, and 41% blastocyst rates [33]. When freezing cleavage-stage embryos on day 2 with the slow freezing method, the survival rate of 77.0% was reported in a study by Xue et al.; however, when using vitrification, the authors reported 96.6% survival rate when $P < 0.05$ [34]. A study in 2015 documented the survival rate of 96.95% after vitrification of day 3 embryos, in contrast to the 69.06% of the embryos survived after slow freezing, post-warmed excellent morphology embryos: 94.17 vs. 60.8% [35]. The study included 592 frozen/thawed embryos. Regarding blastocyst cryopreservation, a large retrospective study by Richter et al. in 2016 included 4862 slow frozen blastocysts and 2735 vitrified blastocysts, with no statistical difference between patients BMI and age [36], and reported interesting findings. A survival rate (authors define survival as having >50% of cells intact after thawing) of 95.6% was achieved in the vitrification group versus 91.9% in the slow frozen group, when $P < .0001$. They also found that the percentage of intact cells was more after vitrification/warming compared to slow freezing and thawing, 95.3 vs. 88.7%, $P < .0001$. It is important to mention that currently, there is much debate as to the developmental stage at which human embryos are best to be cryopreserved [24, 37].

In 2014, a population-based cohort study in Australia and New Zealand included 11,644 slow frozen and thawed blastocysts and 19,978 vitrified and thawed blastocysts. A higher clinical pregnancy rate per embryo transfer cycle was reported for the vitrification group (32.7%) than in the slow frozen one (23.8%). The mean maternal age for the slow frozen group was 33.6, while for the vitrification group—34.2. This is one of the largest known studies in this field; however, a possible drawback could be the lack of information available on clinic-specific cryopreservation protocols and processes for slow freezing-thawing and vitrification-warming of blastocysts and the potential impact on outcomes [38].

All of these results highlight the advantages of vitrification and the drawbacks of slow freezing. Overall, vitrification turns out to be the better method of cryopreservation in the field of ART.

3.3 Consequences of freezing an embryo

There are two major concerns regarding embryo cryopreservation. One of them is about the survival rate after embryo freezing. The second major concern is that the freezing process may induce cryodamage to the embryo. Cryodamage is a collective term which includes various types of injuries that a biological object could experience during the freezing and thawing, like formation of ice crystals, physical stress, and also other types of damage we have mentioned earlier. Assessing survival rate after thawing is the most used technique to evaluate the effects of the cryopreservation process on the embryos. However, freezing an embryo also does not allow the inspection of other types of damages, which occur at the molecular level—DNA damage, altered gene expression, and protein function. These alterations require specific molecular biology methods in order to be assessed, and their impact on the embryo is not that clear. In contrast, when the survival rate after freezing is being assessed, we must say that this approach is straightforward and yields distinct results.

When talking about the embryo survival rate nowadays, with the constantly improving cryopreservation techniques, a survival rate of more than 90% or even 95% could be observed depending on the vitrification protocol, carrier, embryologist experience, thawing process, and other variables. While this rate is indeed very high, unfortunately there is still a risk that a frozen embryo would not survive after thawing. The survival rate is different for the different stages at which the embryos are frozen. In fact, it is still unknown at which stage of development, the embryos are most suitable for freezing and therefore further research is needed. Moreover, the stage at which the embryo is frozen is connected to different types of cryodamage. At the PN stage, there is evidence that embryos may suffer integrity damage of the pronuclei after cryopreservation [39], and therefore, their developmental potential could be significantly impaired. At the cleavage stage, there is evidence of zona pellucida damage [40] and changes in metabolism [41]. Reduced implantation rates have been observed after the loss of blastomeres in day 2 grade 1 embryos with <10% fragmentation in a study with 363 thawing cycles [42]. Blastocyst cryopreservation represents a demanding task due to its size and the presence of blastocoel. Formation of ice crystals is probably the main factor affecting blastocysts survival rates, since the blastocoel contains large amounts of water. In order to reduce the negative effects of the blastocoel on survival rates, it was proposed that blastocysts should be frozen at the contraction stage or the blastocoel should be collapsed artificially before freezing [43] which can be done, for example, with an ICSI pipette. Despite all these difficulties, blastocyst survival rates seem to be higher compared to early cleavage embryos, as shown in a study by Cobo et al., where 6019 embryos were vitrified using Cryotop as a carrier [44]. In the study, 97.6% day 6 embryos survived compared to 95.7% day 5 embryos, 94.9% day 2, and 94.2% day 3 embryos. As a consequence of the freezing procedure, zona pellucida may become thicker, which could affect the implantation ability of the embryo, and this is why assisted hatching is performed with the idea to overcome this problem.

3.4 Artificial shrinkage

In a well expanded blastocyst, the large blastocoel may interfere with the permeation of CPAs during the vitrification procedure which in turn would decrease the survival rates after thawing. Mukaida et al. back in 2003 stated that blastocyst survival rate after vitrification/warming correlate negatively with the expansion of the blastocoel [45]. Artificial shrinkage (AS) of the blastocoel by different methods—laser pulse, microneedle, micropipetting, and 29-gauge needle was developed with the idea of overcoming this obstacle. A study by Gala et al. in 2014 encompassing 185 warming cycles reported a higher survival rate after AS (99.0%) compared to 91.8% survival rate in the control group without AS [46]. Darwish and Magdi in 2016 assessed clinical pregnancy rates, implantation rates, and blastocyst survival rates in more than 400 patients, divided into two groups—untreated expanded blastocysts and blastocysts undergone AS by laser pulse [47]. The study group found that after AS, there was significantly increased survival rates (97.3 vs. 74.9%), implantation (39.1 vs. 24.5%), and clinical pregnancy rates (67.2 vs. 41.1%).

Despite the promising results of AS, this technique is relatively new and not well studied. More studies must be carried out to validate if the procedure is safe and to assess its impact on the developing embryo. Moreover, a high survival rate can be obtained without AS, and therefore, the use of AS is questionable.

4. Embryo cryopreservation and ART

All of the advances that had been made in the last two decades regarding embryo cryopreservation would be of no significance if the success rates after FET were minimal. So what is the place of embryo cryopreservation among other basic ART methods? What are the positives and negatives of having embryos frozen/thawed and transferred instead of having a fresh transfer? We will try to give answers to these very important questions.

4.1 Embryo storage

The main indication of embryo cryopreservation is for storage purposes. We have reviewed the basic cryopreservation methods. Our interpretation of this thought is: however, no matter how much they have improved recently, they could not be successful unless proper storage and thawing of the frozen objects are carried out. After freezing, the embryos are placed in storage tanks which are filled with liquid nitrogen. There is substantial variety of storage tanks and automated storage systems have been recently introduced, which offer optimal storage conditions and safety. It is not known for how long embryos can be stored in liquid nitrogen without affecting their potential, because embryo freezing was developed during the 1980s, which means that the longest time an embryo has been stored is around 35 years, and there is little chance that patients would come back for them after such a long period. There are some differences in the laws regarding embryo cryopreservation, and therefore, embryo storage limit varies between countries, for example, 3 years in Portugal, 5 years in Denmark, Norway, and many other countries, 10 years in Austria and Australia, 55 years in the UK, while in Venezuela, embryo freezing is prohibited [48]. However, a storage time of 5–10 years is most commonly observed.

Keeping embryos in liquid nitrogen raises some concerns about the safety of the procedure. First of all, liquid nitrogen that is used by the IVF laboratories has chemical standards of purity, not biological. That means that there might be some kind of contamination and we should think if there is any way to sterilize this liquid nitrogen. Bielanski et al. describes the potential for viral transmission from experimentally contaminated liquid nitrogen to vitrified embryos, stored in open freezing containers [49]. From a pool of 83 batches, 21% were positive for viral association. In contrast, vitrified embryos in sealed plastic cryovials and straws were free from viral contamination. These data support that sealing of the freezing container might prevent exposure to contaminants; however, that does not mean 100% safety, as the seal can be damaged. This information leads us back to the idea of sterilizing the liquid nitrogen. However, if this is possible, it should be evaluated if it can be applied practically.

Regarding the thawing process, it is very similar in both vitrification and slow freezing technique. The idea is to submerge the frozen object into a solution prewarmed at 37°C which is the core temperature in human body. Closed systems are usually plunged into water baths, while open systems could be put directly into a prewarmed medium. As mentioned before, CPAs are used for the cryopreservation of embryos and those CPAs must be removed during the thawing process and also the cells must be rehydrated. This happens by incubating the embryo in decreasing concentrations of the CPAs and increasing concentrations of water.

4.2 Embryo freezing in clinical practice

Increasing the reliability of the embryo freezing/thawing procedure has enabled a wider application of the method in assisted reproduction.

Indications to why we freeze embryos and do not switch to fresh ET are: OHSS risk and significant increase in progesterone on the day of HCG administration during stimulation. Progesterone levels above 1.5 ng/ml in patients in advanced reproductive age are associated with lower success rates with fresh ET [50], low responders, inadequacy of the cervix, requiring hysteroscopy, areas affected with Zika virus, or the analysis of endometrial implantation “window.”

When patients have cryopreserved embryos it provides them with additional embryo transfers thus increasing the chances of achieving a pregnancy from a single stimulated cycle. This also means that further cycles of hormonal stimulation are not required. Having supernumerary embryos frozen also facilitates the so-called single embryo transfer which helps in avoiding multiple pregnancies. Additionally, freezing of embryos enables patients to decide when is the most appropriate time to start their conceiving efforts.

For patients suffering from cancer, embryos can be frozen before the patient starts cancer treatment, which is done because chemotherapy may negatively affect one’s reproductive ability, and this may be their only option of having offspring.

Freezing embryos also gives the opportunity for genetic testing (PGD/PGS) which is essential in couples with recurrent pregnancy loss and older women who possess higher risk for chromosomal abnormalities.

The frozen embryos may be donated for scientific purposes or they may be used in a donor program if permitted by law, which is also an advantage.

Embryo cryopreservation has many benefits; however, there are some potential risks, and we hope that they will be eliminated in the near future, as this area of research is further developed.

5. Present and future perspectives

Looking at SART statistics, we can find that the number of frozen embryo transfers has increased more than 2.5 times over the 2004/2013 period. Accordingly, for 2004, we have 15,474 frozen embryo transfers vs. 40,015 FETs for 2013, while the number of fresh embryo transfers remains relatively unchanged, respectively, for 2004—2087,089 fresh ET and 87,045 for 2013. On the other hand, there has been a significant increase in the success rate of FET compared to fresh ET. In 2004, the average success rate of FET was 27.8%, while that of fresh ET was at 33%. In 2013, the average success rate of FET was 40.1% and of fresh ET it was 36.3% [51]. Another interesting fact supporting the increased success rate of FET is data from the Japanese National Registry on the number of ART procedures and their success rate based on births. The most significant is in 2014 when the children born after ART were 47,292, with 77.4% of them being after FET [52].

But when discussing frozen embryos and their clinical practice use, the first question arising is the risk to the offspring, when we are applying that technology. The risk for at least one major congenital abnormality of the children born after FET was not increased compared to the children born after fresh ET [53]. On the contrary, the increase in blastogenesis birth defects appears greater for fresh ET than for FET, and the frequency of Down syndrome was statistically more likely in the children born after fresh ET than FET [54]. On the other hand, FET has advantages in that it decreases the risk of low birth weight (LBW) (<2500 g), very low birth weight (<1500 g), very preterm birth (VPTB) (<32 gw), placenta previa, small, placental abruption, gestational age, antepartum hemorrhage, ectopic pregnancy, and perinatal mortality [55, 56]. If we look at the weight indicator of the newborn after ART, the results of the studies show that ART-born children have a lower weight, and the risk of LBW in newborns is 2.6 higher than those spontaneously conceived [57]. However, after FET, children are being born 90–190 g heavier than those after fresh ET. This brings them statistically closer to the children born after a spontaneous pregnancy [54, 58].

Here a question arises: is the change in the weight of the newborn due to epigenetic reprogramming?

Human studies have shown that different ART methods, such as ovarian stimulation and supraphysiological levels of sex steroid hormones, culture media, and embryo cryopreservation, may be associated with intrauterine growth change, resulting in altered birth weight profiles, which may be caused by epigenetic modifications [59]. Furthermore, some reports indicate that children conceived by ART have an altered lipid profile, fasting glucose, body fat distribution, and cardiovascular function [60, 61]. ICSI/IVF children showed a significantly decreased DNA methylation at birth. Studies suggest an impact of ICSI on the offspring's epigenome(s), which may contribute to phenotypic variation and disease susceptibility in ART children [62].

Differences in DNA methylation between IVF and non-IVF twins on a genome-wide scale and their results show evidence for epigenetic modifications that may in part reflect parental subfertility [63].

The methylation profiles of ART and IUI newborns were different from those of naturally conceived newborns. But the profiles of ICSI-frozen (FET) and IUI infants were very similar, suggesting that cryopreservation may eliminate some of the epigenetic aberrations induced by IVF or ICSI [64].

In addition to the above mentioned advantages, frozen ET, compared to fresh ET, also has some drawbacks, such as: macrosomia (OR 1.64), large for gestation age (OR 1.54), post-term birth (OR 1.40), and placenta accrete (OR 3.20) [65]. In cases with preeclampsia, the risk after FET in twin pregnancies is 19.6% with risk difference 5.1% in fresh ET, while in singleton pregnancies, the risk is 7.0% after FET with risk difference 1.8% in fresh ET [66]. Probably, the main reason for the increase of these complications is the protocol of the endometrium preparation for FET. Analyzing the Japanese assisted reproductive technology registry in 2014, Saito et al. [67] found that pregnancies following FET after hormone replacement cycle (n = 75,474 cases) have significant higher risks of hypertensive disorders and placenta accrete compared to FET in natural ovulatory cycle (n = 29,760 cases).

Due to the many advantages of FET compared to fresh ET, a number of clinics have begun to implement the "freeze all" policy, so they do not perform ET in the stimulated cycle, but rather freeze all embryos. In a subsequent or later cycle, with or without HRT (hormone replacement therapy), the embryos are thawed, and ET is performed.

The first publications of results show optimism, because the FET success rate is significantly higher than that of the classic ET approach. In support of these results, it was reported by Lopez et al. in a retrospective study with 1697 IVF cycles that the FET versus fresh ET rate for women up to 39 years was 44.5–38% and for women after 39 years, 34.9% and 22.7%, respectively [68].

Similar results were presented from another retrospective study made by Santistevan et al. [69]. It encompassed more than 16,000 IVF cases, with

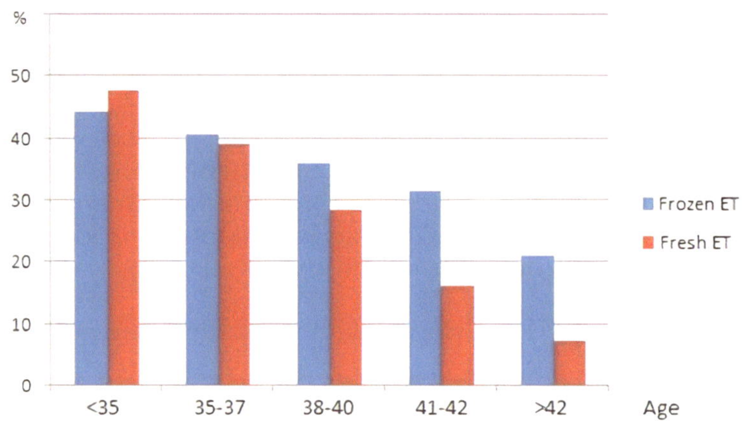

Figure 2.
Age characteristics and fertility in nondonor IVF program after ET of fresh and thawed embryos (SART 2013).

repeated success rates following FET versus fresh ET in women up to 35 years of age, being 50.240.3%. In women after the age of 35, the ratio was 46–33%, respectively. Another interesting study was published by Zhu et al. [70], which included 20,687 women who started their first IVF cycles using a "freeze-all" strategy. The authors report an average success rate of 50.74% live birth rates, establishing different success rates depending on collected oocytes and the age of the woman.

However, despite these preliminary positive results, it must be emphasized that these are retrospective studies. We cannot find enough proof to convince us to change our treatment strategy toward a "freeze all" policy, as the studies cannot give us an answer when it is better to freeze the embryos and when to apply fresh ET.

For this reason, a number of prospective studies are currently being carried out which are intended to answer those questions. What is the place of "freeze all" policy in treatment of infertility? Some of these studies have already published their results, such as Coates et al., who for the first time compared the success rate of FET to that of fresh ET of euploid embryos. In a study encompassing 179 cases, the authors found a significant increase in the success rate of frozen ET, based on developing pregnancy and delivery [71].

In another prospective study, however, Vuong et al. [72] and Shi et al. [73] did not establish a statistically significant difference between FET and fresh ET. The results in the first study were 36.3 and 34.5% in 782 IVF/ICSI cases of non-PCOS patients, while in the second study, the results were 48.7 and 50.2%, respectively, in 2157 women who were undergoing their first in vitro fertilization cycle. The main conclusions of those articles are that freezing embryos do not decrease pregnancy rates, and the "freeze all" policy only raises expenses. But there were some limitations to those studies. The methodology is based on the embryo cultivation to an early cleavage stage, and if the effect of the freezing procedure is sought, the embryos should be cultured and frozen during the blastocyst phase. In support of that opinion is the analysis of the success rates of 236,191 cases after FET. Holden et al. [74] found that there is a 49% increase of live births after blastocyst-stage FET, compared to cleavage-stage FET. The authors examined only a group of patients up to 35 years of age. However, if we were to analyze the success rate after in vitro procedures in different age groups, we would find that in females more than 37 years of age, the results after frozen transfer are significantly higher than in fresh transfer [51] (**Figure 2**).

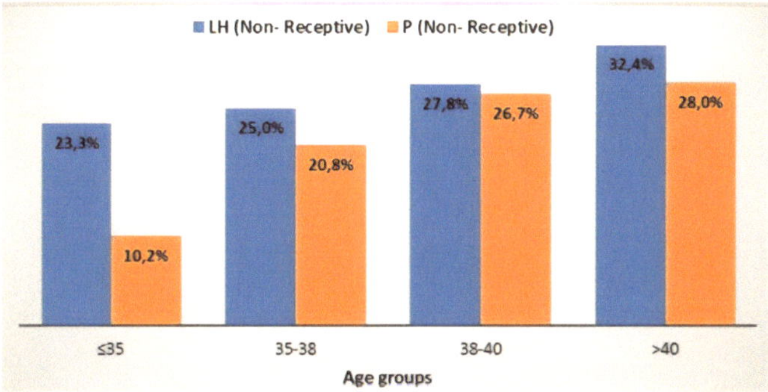

Figure 3.
Age distribution of cases with endometrial non-receptivity (endometrial receptivity analysis) in LH/HRT protocols.

In spite of controversial results, FET has its own place in treatment of couples with infertility. To date, the main explanation for the high FET success rate is the so-called "Hormonal Theory." According to it, high levels of estrogen during stimulation have a detrimental effect on embryos and placentation, a negative effect on the preparation of the endometrium for implantation of the embryo. If we accept this hypothesis, we would not be able to explain why women in advanced reproductive age achieve FETs with higher success rates than fresh ET. The results of the studies show that, as women age, there is a higher possibility of a displacement of the implantation "window." In this situation, it is only logical that the FETs have a lower success rate. Continuing the discussion on this issue, Vladimirov et al. [75] researched the age distribution of cases with a displacement of the implantation "window." This is a study with 402 women to whom we have applied the endometrial receptivity analysis (ERA) test due to different indications. The results show that, with the increase of the woman's age, there are increased number of cases of displacement of the implantation "window" with a statistically reliable difference between the groups of up to 35 years and over 42 years (**Figure 3**).

6. Conclusion

According to the "Theory about the Embryo-Cryo treatment," the procedure of freezing/thawing of the embryo probably has a positive "therapeutic" effect on embryos [6]. In fact, results show that FET has a high delivery rate, and the resulting offspring has a better perinatal outcome, compared to children born after fresh ET. The frequency of obstetric complications during pregnancy and children born with congenital abnormalities is lower in FET. However, we still do not have a clear answer to the question, what are the effects of hormonal stimulation and laboratory conditions of cultivation on the normal development and embryo implantation, as well as on pregnancy, birth and development of the individual. These scientific questions and many more still await their answers (**Figure 4**). We believe that applying this freezing approach can reduce the negative effects of the in vitro procedures on embryo development and implantation.

We would like to close this chapter with Mahatma Gandhi's thought: "A nation's greatness is measured by how it treats its weakest members." Our interpretation of this thought is: "The level of human societal development is measured based on how we take care about our unborn children, i.e., the embryos."

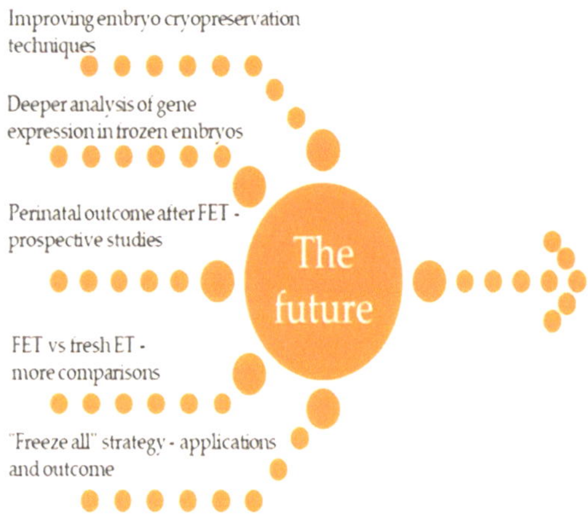

Figure 4.
Possible future directions aiming to improve our understanding of embryo cryopreservation and its place in the field of ART.

Acknowledgements

We would like to express our gratitude to all people who contributed to this work in some way including all the cited authors.

Conflict of interest

None.

Author details

Iavor K. Vladimirov[1,2]*, Desislava Tacheva[1,2] and Vladislav Dobrinov[1]

1 In vitro Fertilization Unit, Sofia Hospital of Obstetrics, Gynaecology and Reproductive Medicine, Sofia, Bulgaria

2 Faculty of Biology, Sofia University "St. Kliment Ohridski", Sofia, Bulgaria

*Address all correspondence to: vladimirov@ivf.bg

References

[1] Woods E, Benson J, Agca Y, Critser J. Fundamental cryobiology of reproductive cells and tissues. Cryobiology. 2004;**48**(2):146-156. DOI: 10.1016/j.cryobiol.2004.03.002

[2] Gosden R. Prospects for oocyte banking and in vitro maturation. Journal of the National Cancer Institute Monographs. 2005;**2005**(34):60-63. DOI: 10.1093/jncimonographs/lgi007

[3] Whittingham D, Leibo S, Mazur P. Survival of mouse embryos frozen to −196 and −269 C. Science. 1972;**178**(4059):411-414. DOI: 10.1126/science.178.4059.411

[4] Wilmut I. The effect of cooling rate, warming rate, cryoprotective agent and stage of development of survival of mouse embryos during freezing and thawing. Life Sciences. 1972;**11**(22):1071-1079. DOI: 10.1016/0024-3205(72)90215-9

[5] Trounson A, Mohr L. Human pregnancy following cryopreservation, thawing and transfer of an eight-cell embryo. Nature. 1983;**305**(5936): 707-709. DOI: 10.1038/305707a0

[6] Vladimirov I, Tacheva D, Diez A. Theory about the embryo cryo-treatment. Reproductive Medicine and Biology. 2017;**16**(2):118-125. DOI: 10.1002/rmb2.12027

[7] Polge C, Smith A, Parkes A. Revival of spermatozoa after vitrification and dehydration at low temperatures. Nature. 1949;**164**(4172):666-666. DOI: 10.1038/164666a0

[8] Isachenko V, Isachenko E, Katkov I, Montag M, Dessole S, Nawroth F, et al. Cryoprotectant-free cryopreservation of human spermatozoa by vitrification and freezing in vapor: Effect on motility, DNA integrity, and fertilization ability. Biology of Reproduction. 2004;**71**(4):1167-1173. DOI: 10.1095/biolreprod.104.028811

[9] Bunge RG, Keettel WC, Sherman JK. Clinical use of frozen semen. Fertility and Sterility. 1954;**5**:520-529. DOI: 10.1016/S0015-0282(16)31802-7

[10] Chen C. Pregnancy after human oocyte cryopreservation. The Lancet. 1986;**327**(8486):884-886. DOI: 10.1016/S0140-6736(86)90989-X

[11] Javed M, Esfandiari N, Swain J, Michael E. Human oocyte cryopreservation—An emerging ART technique: Are we heading in the right direction? Journal of Reproductive Biotechnology and Fertility. 2011;**2**(2):109-120. DOI: 10.1177/205891581100200205

[12] Gook D, Osborn S, Johnston W. Cryopreservation of mouse and human oocytes using 1, 2-propanediol and the configuration of the meiotic spindle. Human Reproduction. 1993;**8**(7):1101-1109. DOI: 10.1093/oxfordjournals.humrep.a138201

[13] Bernard A, Hunter J, Fuller B, Imoedemhe D, Curtis P, Jackson A. Fertilization and embryonic development of human oocytes after cooling. Human Reproduction. 1992;**7**(10):1447-1450. DOI: 10.1093/oxfordjournals.humrep.a137592

[14] Cohen J, Simons R, Edwards R, Fehilly C, Fishel S. Pregnancies following the frozen storage of expanding human blastocysts. Journal of In Vitro Fertilization and Embryo Transfer. 1985;**2**(2):59-64. DOI: 10.1007/bf01139337

[15] Mazur P. Fundamental cryobiology and the preservation of organs by freezing. In: Karow AM, Pegg DE, editors. Organ Preservation for

Transplantation 2nd. New York: Marcel Dekker; 1984. pp. 143-175

[16] Rezazadeh Valojerdi M, Eftekhari-Yazdi P, Karimian L, Hassani F, Movaghar B. Vitrification versus slow freezing gives excellent survival, post warming embryo morphology and pregnancy outcomes for human cleaved embryos. Journal of Assisted Reproduction and Genetics. 2009;**26**(6):347-354. DOI: 10.1007/s10815-009-9318-6

[17] Kasai M, Ito K, Edashige K. Morphological appearance of the cryopreserved mouse blastocyst as a tool to identify the type of cryoinjury. Human Reproduction. 2002;**17**(7):1863-1874. DOI: 10.1093/humrep/17.7.1863

[18] Smith A, Polge C. Survival of Spermatozoa at Low Temperatures. Nature. 1950;**166**(4225):668-669. DOI: 10.1038/166668a0

[19] Fahy G, Wowk B, Wu J, Paynter S. Improved vitrification solutions based on the predictability of vitrification solution toxicity. Cryobiology. 2004;**48**(1):22-35. DOI: 10.1016/j.cryobiol.2003.11.004

[20] Crowe J, Crowe L, Mouradian R. Stabilization of biological membranes at low water activities. Cryobiology. 1983;**20**(3):346-356. DOI: 10.1016/0005-2736(84)90017-8

[21] Aller JF, Alberio RH, Iovannitti B, Cabocevila J. Criopreservación de embriones mamíferos 1ª parte. Características generales de La congelación. Revista de Medicina Veterinaria (Buenos Aires). 1995;**76**(2):132-136

[22] Fuller B, Paynter S. Cryopreservation of mammalian embryos. Methods in Molecular Biology. 2007;**368**:325-339. DOI: 10.1007/978-1-59745-362-2_23

[23] Rall W, Fahy G. Ice-free cryopreservation of mouse embryos at −196°C by vitrification. Nature. 1985;**313**(6003):573-575. DOI: 10.1038/313573a0

[24] Fahy G, MacFarlane D, Angell C, Meryman H. Vitrification as an approach to cryopreservation. Cryobiology. 1984;**21, 4**:407-426. DOI: 1016/0011-2240(84)90079-8

[25] Fahy GM. Vitrification: A new approach to organ cryopreservation. In: Merryman HT, editor. Transplantation—Approaches to Graft Rejection. New York: Alan R Liss; 1986. pp. 305-335

[26] Ali J, Shelton J. Design of vitrification solutions for the cryopreservation of embryos. Reproduction. 1993;**99**(2):471-477. DOI: 10.1530/jrf.0.0990471

[27] Hsieh Y, Tsai H, Chang C, Chang C, Lo H, Lai A. Ultrarapid cryopreservation of human embryos: Experience with 1,582 embryos. Fertility and Sterility. 1999;**72**(2):253-256. DOI: 10.1016/S0015-0282(99)00257-5

[28] Yokota Y. Successful pregnancy following blastocyst vitrification: Case report. Human Reproduction. 2000;**15**(8):1802-1803. DOI: 10.1093/humrep/15.8.1802

[29] Vanderzwalmen P. Vitrification of human blastocysts with the Hemi-Straw carrier: application of assisted hatching after thawing. Human Reproduction. 2003;**18**(7):1504-1511. DOI: 10.1093/humrep/deg298

[30] Li D, Yang D, An J, Jiao J, Zhou Y, Wu Q, et al. Effect of assisted hatching on pregnancy outcomes: a systematic review and meta-analysis of randomized controlled trials. Scientific Reports. 2016;**6**(1). DOI: 10.1038/srep31228

[31] Knudtson J, Failor C, Gelfond J, Goros M, Chang T, Schenken R, et al. Assisted hatching and live births in first-cycle frozen embryo transfers. Fertility and Sterility. 2017;**108**(4):628-634. DOI: 10.1016/j.fertnstert.2017.07.011

[32] Panagiotidis Y, Vanderzwalmen P, Prapas Y, Kasapi E, Goudakou M, Papatheodorou A, et al. Open versus closed vitrification of blastocysts from an oocyte-donation programme: A prospective randomized study. Reproductive Biomedicine Online. 2013;**26**(5):470-476. DOI: 10.1016/j.rbmo.2013.01.016

[33] Kuwayama M, Vajta G, Ieda S, Kato O. Comparison of open and closed methods for vitrification of human embryos and the elimination of potential contamination. Reproductive Biomedicine Online. 2005;**11**(5):608-614. DOI: 10.1016/S1472-6483(10)61169-8

[34] Xue S, Lyu Q, Peng Q, Cao S, Zhou Y, Kuang Y. Vitrification yields superior efficiency of human cleavage-stage embryo cryopreservation versus slow-freezing. Fertility and Sterility. 2010;**94**(4):S119-S120. DOI: 10.1016/j.fertnstert.2010.07.486

[35] Choudhary M, Soni R, Swarankar M, Garg S. Comparison of vitrification and slow freezing for cryopreservation of cleavage stage embryos (Day 3) and its impact on clinical outcome. International Journal of Research in Medical Sciences. 2015;**3**(10): 2751-2756. DOI: 10.18203/2320-6012.ijrms20150826

[36] Richter K, Ginsburg D, Shipley S, Lim J, Tucker M, Graham J, et al. Factors associated with birth outcomes from cryopreserved blastocysts: experience from 4,597 autologous transfers of 7,597 cryopreserved blastocysts. Fertility and Sterility. 2016;**106**(2):354-362.e2. DOI: 10.1016/j.fertnstert.2016.04.022

[37] Liebermann J. More than six years of blastocyst vitrification—What is the verdict? American Journal of Obstetrics and Gynecology. 2011;**5**:14-17

[38] Li Z, Wang Y, Ledger W, Edgar D, Sullivan E. Clinical outcomes following cryopreservation of blastocysts by vitrification or slow freezing: a population-based cohort study. Human Reproduction. 2014;**29**(12):2794-2801. DOI: 10.1093/humrep/deu246

[39] Isachenko V, Todorov P, Dimitrov Y, Isachenko E. Integrity rate of pronuclei after cryopreservation of pronuclear-zygotes as a criteria for subsequent embryo development and pregnancy. Human Reproduction. 2008;**23**(4): 819-826. DOI: 10.1093/humrep/den002

[40] Van den Abbeel E. Zona pellucida damage to human embryos after cryopreservation and the consequences for their blastomere survival and in-vitro viability. Human Reproduction. 2000;**15**(2):373-378. DOI: 10.1093/humrep/15.2.373

[41] Balaban B, Urman B, Ata B, Isiklar A, Larman M, Hamilton R, et al. A randomized controlled study of human Day 3 embryo cryopreservation by slow freezing or vitrification: vitrification is associated with higher survival, metabolism and blastocyst formation. Human Reproduction. 2008;**23**(9): 1976-1982. DOI: 10.1093/humrep/den222

[42] Guerif F. Parameters guiding selection of best embryos for transfer after cryopreservation: A reappraisal. Human Reproduction. 2002;**17**(5): 1321-1326. DOI: 10.1093/humrep/17.5.1321

[43] Chian R, Quinn P. Fertility Cryopreservation. Cambridge: Cambridge University Press; 2010. p. 95

[44] Cobo A, de los Santos M, Castellò D, Gámiz P, Campos P,

Remohí J. Outcomes of vitrified early cleavage-stage and blastocyst-stage embryos in a cryopreservation program: evaluation of 3,150 warming cycles. Fertility and Sterility. 2012;**98**(5):1138-1146.e1. DOI: 10.1016/j.fertnstert.2012.07.1107

[45] Mukaida T. Vitrification of human blastocysts using cryoloops: clinical outcome of 223 cycles. Human Reproduction. 2003;**18**(2):384-391. DOI: 10.1093/humrep/deg047

[46] Gala A, Ferrières A, Assou S, Monforte M, Bringer-Deutsch S, Vintejoux E, et al. Effets de la réduction artificielle du blastocèle avant vitrification en système fermé : étude contrôlée randomisée. Gynécologie Obstétrique & Fertilité. 2014;**42**(11):772-778. DOI: 10.1016/j.gyobfe.2014.09.006

[47] Darwish E, Magdi Y. Artificial shrinkage of blastocoel using a laser pulse prior to vitrification improves clinical outcome. Journal of Assisted Reproduction and Genetics. 2016;**33**(4):467-471. DOI: 10.1007/s10815-016-0662-z

[48] Ory SJ, Devroey P, Banker M, Brinsden P, Buster J, Fiadjoe M, Horton M, Nygren K, Pai H, Le Roux P, Sullivan E. IFFS Surveillance 2013. International Federation of Fertility Societies; 2013. Available from: http://www.iffs-reproduction.org/?page=Surveillance [Accessed: 31-05-2018]

[49] Bielanski A, Nadin-Davis S, Sapp T, Lutze-Wallace C. Viral contamination of embryos cryopreserved in liquid nitrogen. Cryobiology. 2000;**40**(2):110-116

[50] Wang A, Santistevan A, Hunter Cohn K, Copperman A, Nulsen J, Miller B, et al. Freeze-only versus fresh embryo transfer in a multicenter matched cohort study: Contribution of progesterone and maternal age to success rates. Fertility and Sterility. 2017;**108**(2):254-261.e4. DOI: 10.1016/j.fertnstert.2017.05.007

[51] IVF success rate reports 2004-2013. Society for Assisted Reproductive Technology [Website]. Available from: https://www.sartcorsonline.com/rptCSR_PublicMultYear.aspx?ClinicPKID=0 [Accessed: 11-12-2015]

[52] Irahara M, Kuwahara A, Iwasa T, Ishikawa T, Ishihara O, Kugu K, et al. Assisted reproductive technology in Japan: A summary report of 1992-2014 by the Ethics Committee, Japan Society of Obstetrics and Gynecology. Reproductive Medicine and Biology. 2017;**16**(2):126-132. DOI: 10.1002/rmb2.12014

[53] Pelkonen S, Hartikainen A, Ritvanen A, Koivunen R, Martikainen H, Gissler M, et al. Major congenital anomalies in children born after frozen embryo transfer: A cohort study 1995-2006. Human Reproduction. 2014;**29**(7):1552-1557. DOI: 10.1093/humrep/deu088

[54] Yamatoya K, Saito K, Saito T, Kang W, Nakamura A, Miyado M, et al. Birthweights and Down syndrome in neonates that were delivered after frozen-thawed embryo transfer: The 2007-2012 Japan Society of Obstetrics and Gynecology National Registry data in Japan. Reproductive Medicine and Biology. 2017;**16**(2):228-234. DOI: 10.1002/rmb2.12033

[55] Maheshwari A, Pandey S, Shetty A, Hamilton M, Bhattacharya S. Obstetric and perinatal outcomes in singleton pregnancies resulting from the transfer of frozen thawed versus fresh embryos generated through in vitro fertilization treatment: A systematic review and meta-analysis. Fertility and Sterility. 2012;**98**(2):368-377.e9. DOI: 10.1016/j.fertnstert.2012.05.019

[56] Pinborg A, Wennerholm U, Romundstad L, Loft A, Aittomaki K,

Soderstrom-Anttila V, et al. Why do singletons conceived after assisted reproduction technology have adverse perinatal outcome? Systematic review and meta-analysis. Human Reproduction Update. 2012;**19**(2): 87-104. DOI: 10.1093/humupd/dms044

[57] Ombelet W, Martens G, Bruckers L. Pregnant after assisted reproduction: A risk pregnancy is born! 18-years perinatal outcome results from a population-based registry in Flanders, Belgium. Facts, views & visions in ObGyn. 2016 Dec;**8**(4):193-204

[58] Vidal M, Vellvé K, González-Comadran M, Robles A, Prat M, Torné M, et al. Perinatal outcomes in children born after fresh or frozen embryo transfer: A Catalan cohort study based on 14,262 newborns. Fertility and Sterility. 2017;**107**(4):940-947. DOI: 10.1016/j.fertnstert.2017.01.021

[59] Pinborg A, Henningsen A, Loft A, Malchau S, Forman J, Andersen A. Large baby syndrome in singletons born after frozen embryo transfer (FET): Is it due to maternal factors or the cryotechnique? Human Reproduction. 2014;**29**(3):618-627. DOI: 10.1093/humrep/det440

[60] Ceelen M, van Weissenbruch M, Prein J, Smit J, Vermeiden J, Spreeuwenberg M, et al. Growth during infancy and early childhood in relation to blood pressure and body fat measures at age 8-18 years of IVF children and spontaneously conceived controls born to subfertile parents. Human Reproduction. 2009;**24**(11):2788-2795. DOI: 10.1093/humrep/dep273

[61] Scherrer U, Rimoldi S, Rexhaj E, Stuber T, Duplain H, Garcin S, et al. Systemic and pulmonary vascular dysfunction in children conceived by assisted reproductive technologies. Circulation. 2012;**125**(15):1890-1896. DOI: 10.1161/circulationaha.111.071183

[62] El Hajj N, Haertle L, Dittrich M, Denk S, Lehnen H, Hahn T, et al. DNA methylation signatures in cord blood of ICSI children. Human Reproduction. 2017;**32**(8):1761-1769. DOI: 10.1093/humrep/dex209

[63] Castillo-Fernandez J, Loke Y, Bass-Stringer S, Gao F, Xia Y, Wu H, et al. DNA methylation changes at infertility genes in newborn twins conceived by in vitro fertilisation. Genome Medicinc. 2017;**9**(1):1-15. DOI: 10.1186/s13073-017-0413-5

[64] Estill M, Bolnick J, Waterland R, Bolnick A, Diamond M, Krawetz S. Assisted reproductive technology alters deoxyribonucleic acid methylation profiles in bloodspots of newborn infants. Fertility and Sterility. 2016;**106**(3):629-639.e10. DOI: 10.1016/j.fertnstert.2016.05.006

[65] Wennerholm U, Henningsen A, Romundstad L, Bergh C, Pinborg A, Skjaerven R, et al. Perinatal outcomes of children born after frozen-thawed embryo transfer: A Nordic cohort study from the CoNARTaS group. Human Reproduction. 2013;**28**(9):2545-2553. DOI: 10.1093/humrep/det272

[66] Opdahl S, Henningsen A, Tiitinen A, Bergh C, Pinborg A, Romundstad P, et al. Risk of hypertensive disorders in pregnancies following assisted reproductive technology: A cohort study from the CoNARTaS group. Human Reproduction. 2015;**30**(7):1724-1731. DOI: 10.1093/humrep/dev090

[67] Saito K, Kuwahara A, Ishikawa T, Nakasuji T, Miyado M, Miyado K, et al. Pregnancy after frozen-thawed embryo transfer during hormonal replacement cycle is associated with hypertensive disorders of pregnancy and placenta accreta. In: ESHRE Annual meeting; Barcelona; 2018, O-283

[68] Lopez S, Lattes K, Vassena R, Brassesco M, Vernaeve V. Freeze-all in older women: Benefit or loss? Human Reproduction. 2016;**31**(5):14

[69] Santistevan A, Cohn K, Arredondo F, Miller B, Ory S, Leondires M, et al. Multi-center study demonstrates freeze-all IVF protocols are correlated with higher ongoing pregnancy rates in women of advanced maternal age. Human Reproduction. 2016;**31**(102-103):111-112

[70] Zhu Q, Chen Q, Wang L, Lu X, Lyu Q, Wang Y, et al. Live birth rates in the first complete IVF cycle among 20 687 women using a freeze-all strategy. Human Reproduction. 2018;**33**(5): 924-929. DOI: 10.1093/humrep/dey044

[71] Coates A, Kung A, Mounts E, Hesla J, Bankowski B, Barbieri E, et al. Optimal euploid embryo transfer strategy, fresh versus frozen, after preimplantation genetic screening with next generation sequencing: A randomized controlled trial. Fertility and Sterility. 2017;**107, 3**:723-730.e3. DOI: 10.1016/j.fertnstert.2016.12.022

[72] Vuong L, Dang V, Ho T, Huynh B, Ha D, Pham T, et al. IVF transfer of fresh or frozen embryos in women without polycystic ovaries. Obstetrical & Gynecological Survey. 2018;**73**(4):214-215. DOI: 10.1097/01.ogx.0000532004.69352.03

[73] Shi Y, Sun Y, Hao C, Zhang H, Wei D, Zhang Y, et al. Transfer of fresh versus frozen embryos in ovulatory women. The New England Journal of Medicine. 2018;**378**(2):126-136

[74] Holden EC, Kashani BN, Morelli SS, Alderson D, Jindal SK, Ohman-Strickland PA, et al. Improved outcomes after blastocyst-stage frozen-thawed embryo transfers compared with cleavage stage: A society for assisted reproductive technologies clinical outcomes reporting system study. Fertility and Sterility. 2018;**110**(1):89-94.e2. DOI: 10.1016/j.fertnstert.2018.03.033

[75] Vladimirov IK, Tacheva D. Frozen Embryo Transfer—Is it our future? In: 19th World Congress on IVF; Antalya; 2017, O-01

Chapter 9

Effect of Assisted Reproductive Technology (ART) on Babies Born: Compared by IVF Laboratories of Two Countries

Linda Wu, Jinzhou Qin, Dikai Zhang, Minqi Zhang, Suzhen Lu, Jennifer Howell, Timothy J. Gelety and Bin Wu

Abstract

Assisted reproductive technology (ART) has been widely used for infertility treatment, but many people have concern about their baby's health. The objective of this chapter is to provide some detailed data about the effect of ART on human birth babies by analyzing the data from in vitro fertilization (IVF) centers in two countries. All recent records related to a baby's birth including mother's age, gestational days, baby's sex, and birth weight data were collected and analyzed according to fresh or frozen embryo transfer procedure. Normal delivery data without ART were used as control. The result showed that ART patient age is significantly older than non-IVF women; the gestation of fresh and frozen embryo transfer is the same as normal spontaneous conception gestation days, but women pregnant with multiple gestations have shorter gestational period and early birth rate as well as low birth weight; and there is no significant difference in the baby's weight between ART singleton babies and normal conception babies, but male babies weight is more than female babies, and multiple gestation's birth weights are significantly lower than singletons, while frozen embryo transfer babies have significantly heavier birth weight than fresh embryo transfer. Also, the frozen embryo transfer technique may significantly decrease premature birth rate. Thus, frozen embryo transfer may be recommended as a health strategy in ART.

Keywords: in vitro fertilization, frozen embryo transfer, baby birth, outcome

1. Introduction

This year is the 41st anniversary of the first test-tube human birth. In 1978, Dr. Robert Edwards, who won the Nobel Prize a few years ago, became the first physician to create a test-tube baby in a laboratory using an in vitro fertilization (IVF) technique on humans. Since this technique's creation, assisted reproductive technology (ART) has been widely used for the treatment of infertile couples to realize their dream of having a baby. Currently, this technology mainly contains in vitro fertilization (IVF) and its related procedures—intracytoplasmic sperm injection (ICSI), frozen embryo transfer (FET), and preimplantation genetic testing (PGT) including aneuploidies (PGT-A, previously known as PGS), monogenic/single-gene defects (PGT-M, previously known as PGD), and chromosomal structural rearrangements (PGT-SR, previously known as PGD screen or PGS) [Note: New PGT nomenclature announced by the International Committee Monitoring Assisted Reproductive Technologies (CMART) in collaboration with the American Society for Reproductive Medicine (ASRM), the European Society of Human Reproduction and Embryology (ESHRE), and other professional medical societies (2018).] [1]. So far, more than 10 million IVF/ICSI and frozen embryo transfer babies have been born throughout the world. This technique indeed brings many infertile families happiness. However, the key point of the assisted reproductive techniques is that the patient needs to be injected with some medicine to stimulate the ovaries to produce more oocytes during one reproductive period cycle and the retrieved oocytes need to be fertilized under an in vitro environment, such as a laboratory. As more infants are born through this technique, there are concerns of whether fertilizing a female egg outside the human body will lead to any negative outcomes on the infant or the mother. For example, if a baby is born through IVF technique, will he or she be at an increased risk for any defects, or will an IVF baby have the same birthweight as a baby conceived naturally? Thus, many people have worried about ART neonatal health outcomes. Recently, many scientists, physicians, general practitioners, reproductive medicine experts, and social media all had a public debut together in Chicago to discuss the birth of the first IVF baby [2]. In early 2005, Bower and Hansen [3] published an overview for assisted reproductive technologies and birth outcomes based on systematic reviews and meta-analyses of randomized controlled trials which included perinatal mortality, preterm birth, low birthweight, and birth defects. In recent years, many IVF centers have reported the IVF baby birth outcome [4]. Overall, they showed that few differences between outcomes in ART twins compared with twins conceived spontaneously, but in singleton pregnancies, ART infants had twofold increases in risk of perinatal mortality, low birthweight and preterm birth, shortened gestational age, and increased birth defects [3]. In November 2005, the *Fertility and Sterility* journal published seven papers related to IVF increased birth defect, and all these studies indicated that ART techniques really increased some risk of birth defects [5–11].

In spite of ART resulting in some birth defects, in the past decade, many assisted reproductive centers have been built throughout the world, and more and more babies have been conceived by assisted reproductive technologies because these techniques provide many infertile couples the opportunity to have a child in their family. Thus, when we use these assisted reproductive technologies to treat infertility, we should concern more current birth baby situation. Currently, many articles and some reviews of ART effects on babies born have reported, but it is very difficult to find systematic data about ART outcomes on sex ratio and the effect of frozen embryo transfer. The objective of this study is to provide detailed data about the effect of ART on babies born by comparing data of two assisted reproductive centers from two different countries.

2. Materials and methods

2.1 Data source

In the USA, based on the reported Society for Assisted Reproductive Technology (SART) data of the Arizona Center for Reproductive Endocrinology and Infertility from 2010 to 2014, all records related to baby births including mother's age, gestational days, baby sex, and birthweight were collected and analyzed according to fresh or frozen embryo transfer procedures. A total of 519 babies were born from 411 mothers from fresh embryo transfer or frozen-thawed embryo transfer techniques. Normal conception data without undergoing ART was also collected from a local obstetrical hospital as control (Tucson Medical Center).

In China, according to delivery records of the Obstetrical Department in Luohu Hospital of Shenzhen City, all data related to baby births including the mother's age, gestational days, sex, and birthweight and length were collected based on fresh or frozen embryo transfer procedures and natural conception delivery situations. A total of 856 babies were born from 657 mothers from fresh embryo transfer or frozen-thawed embryo transfer techniques. Normal conception delivery data without undergoing ART were also collected on babies from 265 mothers at the same obstetrical hospital as control.

2.2 Data classification

For the purpose of this analysis, all ART procedure includes IVF or ICSI treatment and FET data. Characteristics of infants in IVF and FET and control populations may be defined as different groups based on Helmerhorst et al. report [12]: gestation days as preterm (<37 weeks or 259 days) birth, very preterm (<32 weeks or 224 days) birth, and full-term birth and birthweight as low birthweight (<2500 g), very low birthweight (<1500 g), and normal birthweight.

2.3 Data analysis

The average and standard deviation (means) of all data were calculated by Microsoft Excel Ware. The significant differences between the averages were examined by student t-test statistical analysis, the baby sex ratio difference was examined by $\chi 2$ test, and the difference between the percentages was examined by percentage test method. The differences were considered statistically significant at $P < 0.05$.

3. Results

Based on the analysis of the Arizona center data, the summary of birth information is listed in **Table 1**.

From this table, we may see some important points on outcomes of ART babies:

A. Women undergoing ART with fresh embryo transfer and frozen embryo transfer are significantly older than women with normal conception women ($P < 0.05$), while the ages of women with multiple conception are significantly younger than normal ART procedures but older than women with natural pregnancy ($P < 0.05$).

B. The gestational days following fresh embryo transfer are similar to babies born naturally (269.6 vs. 272.2 days, $P > 0.05$), but women with multiple gestations have a shorter gestation period (240 days, $P < 0.01$), and frozen embryo transfer women have a slightly longer gestation period (273 days, $P < 0.05$), but it did not have significant difference with normal conception infant (272.2 vs. 273 days, $P > 0.05$).

	Fresh IVF/ICSI single birth	Frozen embryo transfer single birth	Multiple births (twin/triplet)	Normal delivery birth
Patient no.	235	78	98	95
Patient age	33.84 ± 4.96[a] 20–45	34.59 ± 4.11[a] 24–45	32.95 ± 4.60[b] 22–43	27.93 ± 5.68[c]
Gestation days	269.57 ± 13.28[a] 211–297	273.00 ± 11.12[b] 234–293	239.60 ± 27.46[c]	272.16 ± 8.8[a,b]
Male no.*	126	36	100	47
Female no.	109	42	106	48
Male birthweight (g)	3227.71 ± 587.06[a] 1470–4706	3401 ± 479.81[b] 2637–4621	2242.21 ± 598.98[c] 680–3402	3310.21 ± 461.88[b]
Female birthweight (g)	3005.36 ± 427.15[d] 1250–4337	3229 ± 423.34[a] 2070–4163	2046.97 ± 654.98[e] 482–3317	3188.5 ± 424.86[a]
Total birthweight (g)	3122 ± 530.28[a] 1250–4706	3308.83 ± 453.25[b] 2070–4621	2133.17 ± 631.88[c] 482–3402	3248.72 ± 445.41[b] 2040–4690
<1500 g (%)	0.85	0	17	1.05
<2500 g (%)	11.50	3.85	67.96	4.21
Full-term birth (%)	86.81	92.31	27.83	94.73
Preterm (%)	11.49[a]	7.69[b]	51.76[c]	5.27
Very preterm	1.7	0	20.41	0
Multiple rate	25.39	18.75		3.00

The different small letters indicate significant difference (P<0.05).

Table 1.
Summary for birth outcomes from various ART procedures of the Arizona IVF Center.

C. Based on gestational day analysis, there is no significant difference on very preterm birth (<224 days) or preterm delivery (<259 days) between fresh embryo transfer, frozen embryo transfer singletons, and normal deliveries (13.19 vs. 13.91%, $P > 0.05$), but multiple gestations have significantly higher preterm birth rate (72%), and frozen embryo transfer has lower early birth rate (7.69%, $P < 0.01$).

D. After χ^2 test, there is no significant difference in the incidence of male or female babies although fresh embryo transfer had a trend of more male babies (53.6%) and frozen embryo transfer had more female babies (53.8%).

E. Based on birthweight comparison, there is a significant difference among the singleton infant of fresh embryo transfer, frozen embryo transfer, and normal normally conceived babies ($P < 0.05$). The fresh embryo transfer infants have lower birthweight than frozen embryo transfer and normally conceived babies, but there is no difference between the frozen embryo transfer and natural conception babies. Also, male infant birthweight is heavier than female infant birthweight (3227 vs. 3005 g, $P < 0.05$), and multiple gestation birthweights are significantly less than singletons (2242 vs. 3227 g, $P < 0.05$), while frozen embryo transfer babies have significantly heavier birthweights than fresh embryo transfer (3401 vs. 3227 g, $P < 0.01$). Meanwhile we have found that 11.5% infants of fresh transfer singletons have less 2500 g birthweight, which is a significantly higher rate than frozen embryo transfer and natural conception babies. Further, 68% of multiple gestations have a very low birthweight.

F. The rate of multiple gestational births is significantly higher in ART group than the natural conception group.

Based on the China ART center data (**Table 2**), the following several points may be observed.

From this table, we may observe the following important points:

a. Patients undergoing ART are significantly older than natural conception patients.

b. The gestational days of singleton following fresh embryo transfer and frozen-thawed embryo transfer are similar to babies born from natural conception (268 vs. 270 days, $P > 0.05$), but multiple gestations have a shorter gestation period (253 or 251 days, $P < 0.01$). Based on gestational day analysis, there is no significant difference on preterm birth (<259 days) or full-term birth among fresh embryo transfer, frozen embryo transfer singletons, and natural conception babies ($P > 0.05$), but multiple gestations have a significantly higher preterm birth rate (41%) with fresh and frozen-thawed embryo transfer (52%, $P < 0.01$).

c. Based on total birthweight comparison, there is no significant difference on the baby weight among the singleton infants of fresh embryo transfer, frozen embryo transfer, and normal conception babies ($P > 0.05$). However, the male babies with fresh and frozen-thawed embryos have a heaver birthweight than female babies ($P < 0.05$), but there is no difference between the male and female birthweights with natural conception babies. The multiple birthweights are significantly less than singletons ($P < 0.05$), while frozen embryo transfer

	Fresh IVF/ ICSI single birth	**Frozen ET single birth**	**Multiple birth (fresh ET)**	**Multiple birth (frozen ET)**	**Naturally delivered baby birth**
Patient no.	251	207	100	99	265
Patient age	33.7 ± 3.7^{a}	34.8 ± 4.2^{a}	32.2 ± 3.8^{a}	33.1 ± 3.2^{a}	27.2 ± 3.0^{b}
Gestation days	268.2 ± 11^{a} 231–294	268.1 ± 14^{a} 189–287	253 ± 12^{b} 210–273	251 ± 14^{b} 182–273	270.6 ± 16^{a} 235–289
Male no.	120	116	108	115	139
Female no.	131	91	94	81	126
Male birthweight (g)	$3314 \pm 560^{a,A}$ 2000–4900	$3353 \pm 474.76^{a,A}$ 1150–5900	2431 ± 382^{b} 1250–3250	$2537 \pm 393^{b,A}$ 1150–3600	3200 ± 600^{a} 1550–4850
Female birthweight (g)	$3140 \pm 510^{a,B}$ 1790–4300	$3215 \pm 423.34^{a,B}$ 1600–4200	2423 ± 381^{b} 1500–3500	$2433 \pm 461^{b,B}$ 930–3400	3200 ± 500^{a} 1750–4750
Total	3223.40 ± 476^{a} 1790–4900	3292.44 ± 557^{a} 1150–5900	2474.18 ± 398^{b} 1250–3650	2493.8 ± 442^{b} 930–3600	3200 ± 550^{a} 1550–4850
Full-term birth (%)	88.05^{a}	87.98^{a}	59.0^{b}	47.48^{b}	89.2^{a}
Early birth (%)	11.95^{a}	12.02^{a}	41.0^{b}	52.52^{b}	10.8^{a}

The different small letters indicate row significant difference, and the different capital letters indicate column significant difference.

Table 2.
Summary of birth outcomes from the Chinese Luohu IVF Center.

babies have slightly heavier birthweight than fresh embryo transfer (3292 vs. 3223 g, $P < 0.05$).

d. Based on sex ratio analysis, there is a significant difference between the numbers of male and female infants in ART babies ($P < 0.05$). In general, there are more male than female babies (53.6 vs. 46.4%) in ART, which is similar to natural conception births (52.5 vs. 47.5%). However, the fresh embryo transfer showed less male than female babies (47.8 vs. 52.2%). In the frozen embryo transfer program, male babies were significantly higher than female babies (56 vs. 44%). In natural conception babies, although there is no statistically significant difference between sex ratio, 52.5% are male babies and 47.5% are female babies.

4. Discussion

Forty years ago, the first baby was born by IVF. So far, thousands of human IVF centers or clinics have been set up, and hundreds and thousands of IVF babies have been born all over the world [13–16]. This technology has brought many infertile families happiness. However, there has been a concern as to the safety of this technology and the health of the babies. Currently, many reports have shown that there is no clear evidence that these babies are more at risk from abnormalities than those born through natural conception. Indeed, it seems that certain types of abnormalities, such as chromosomal problems, are less common with IVF, but IVF babies tend to have more problems at birth, and stillbirth may be slightly more common. This may not be due to IVF technological problem, and it is probably because women who conceive through IVF are more likely to be at high risk in pregnancy. Different countries or different IVF centers often report various outcomes. In order to get a common knowledge of IVF's influence on birth, our study compared the outcomes of two different IVF laboratories in two different countries. The comparative results showed that the ages of patients undergoing IVF are significantly older than normal conception in both countries (**Figure 1**). This is mainly due to problems with infertility. Many patients tried to conceive by natural methods for many years, but they did not get pregnancy. Thus, these patients' final hope was to undergo IVF to resolve their problems. This often results in some high-risk complications due to the advancing age.

Figure 2 showed that the gestational days of two laboratories following fresh embryo transfer are similar to babies conceived naturally, but multiple gestations have a shorter gestational period (240 days at the Arizona center and 252 days at the Luohu center). The Arizona center had less gestational days because it had more triplets than the Luohu center, which had more twin gestations.

The gestational day analysis also showed that there is no significant difference on very preterm birth (<224 days) or preterm delivery (<259 days) between fresh embryo transfer, frozen embryo transfer singletons, and normal conceptions, but multiple gestations have significantly higher preterm birth rate, and frozen embryo transfer has lower preterm birth rate (**Figures 3** and **4**). The frozen embryo transfer showed a similar full-term birth to natural conception pregnancies (92 vs. 94%). Recently a meta-analysis confirmed that singleton babies conceived by frozen embryo transfers are at lower risk of preterm delivery, small for gestational age, and low birthweight, but it may increase risks of large for gestational age and macrosomia [17, 18]. Also, researchers from the USA found that extremely high estrogen levels at the time of embryo transfer may increase the risk that infants will be born small for their gestational age as well as an increased risk of preeclampsia. They proposed freezing embryos of women who

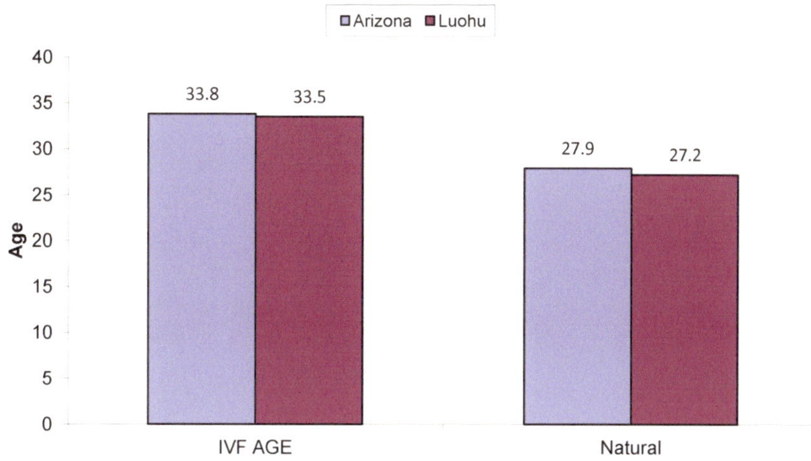

Figure 1.
Age comparison of IVF patients and natural conception patients.

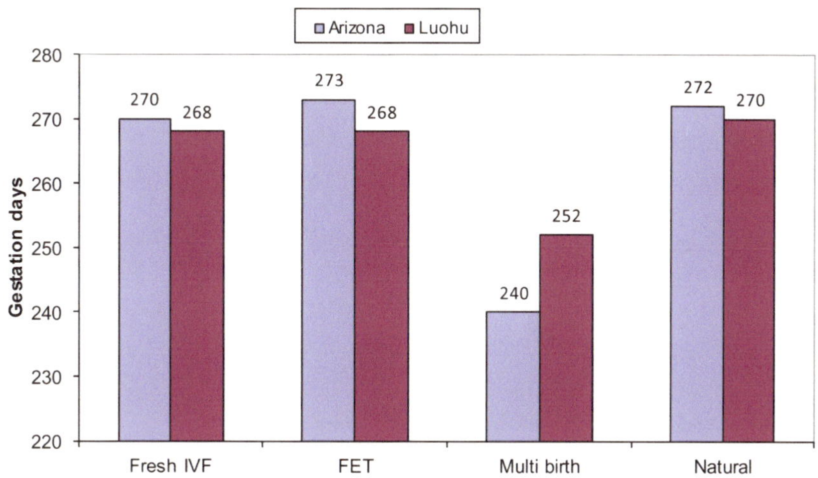

Figure 2.
The comparison of gestational days with various ART procedures.

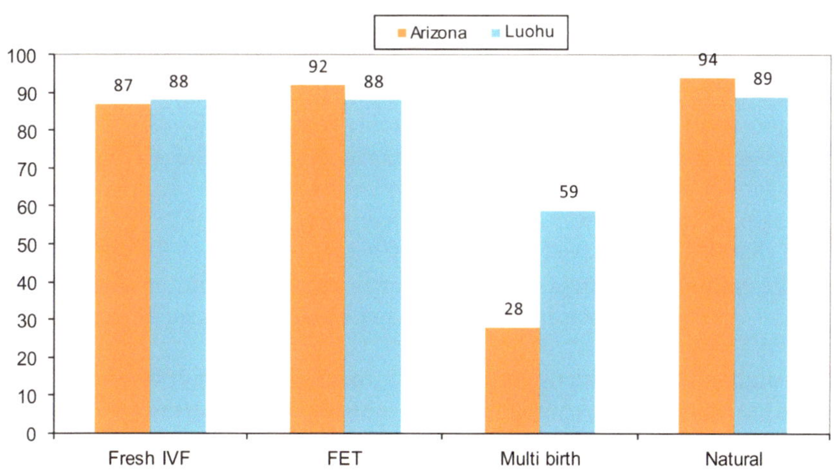

Figure 3.
The comparison of full-term birth percentage in various procedures.

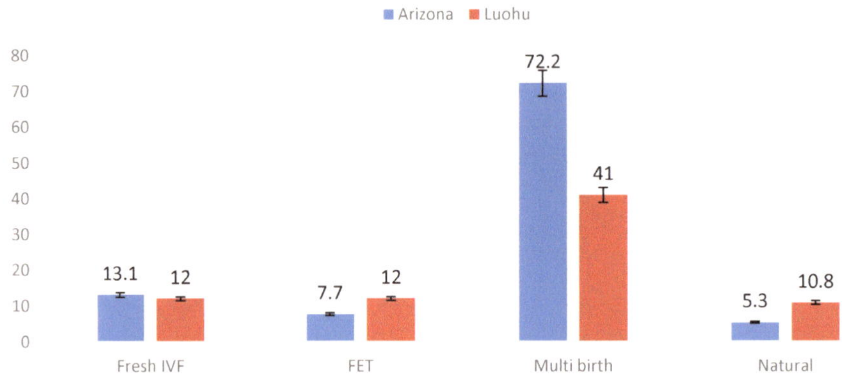

Figure 4.
The percentage of preterm birth with various procedures.

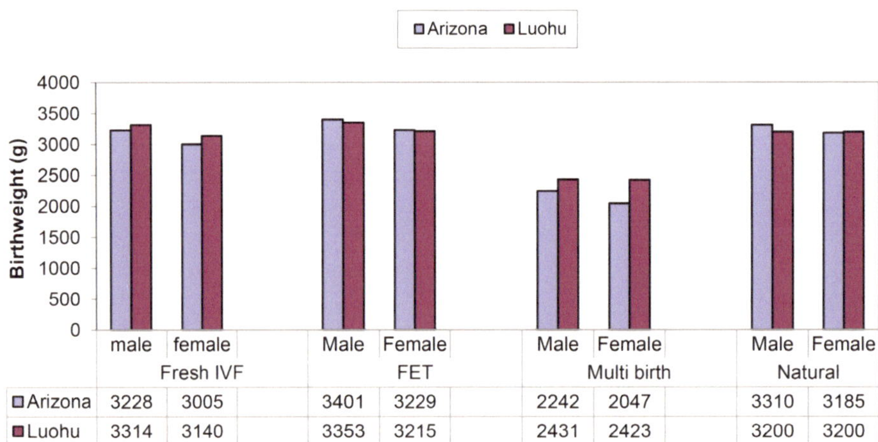

Figure 5.
The birthweight comparison of various procedures in male vs. female.

have excessively elevated estrogen at the time of egg collection, followed by embryo transfer in a later cycle when hormonal levels were closer to those of a natural cycle [17, 19].

Based on the total birthweight comparison (**Figure 5**), there is no significant difference on the baby weight among the singleton infants of fresh embryo transfer, frozen embryo transfer, and normal conception babies in the Luohu center. The fresh embryo transfer infants have a lower birthweight than frozen embryo transfer and natural conception babies in Luohu, but there is no difference between the frozen embryo transfer and natural conception babies at the Arizona center. Recently, a meta-analysis confirmed that singleton babies conceived by frozen embryo transfer were at lower risk than fresh embryo transfer [19, 20]. These results indicated that IVF technique shows no big effect on singleton IVF birth. However, multiple gestation birthweights are significantly less than singletons in the two laboratories. Further analysis indicated that male babies are heavier than female babies in all IVF groups.

According to sex ratio analysis, two laboratories displayed different results (**Figure 6**). At the Arizona center, the fresh embryo transfer often produced more male babies. This is due to the selection of fast-growing and good quality embryos on day 3 for transfer. Evidence shows that most of the fast-growing embryos are male [21]. After selection, some slow-growing embryos would be frozen, and after thawing and transfer, they often produce more female embryos. However, at the

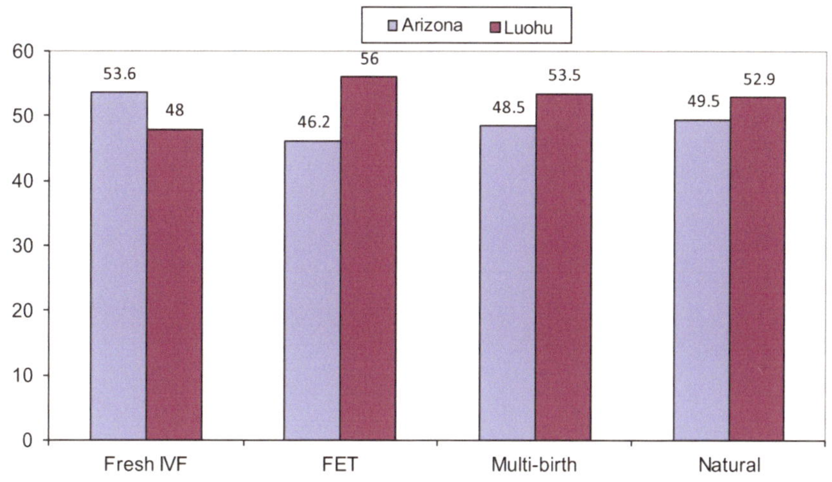

Figure 6.
Male baby percentage of various ART procedures.

Luohu center, their procedure was different from the Arizona center. Fresh embryo transfer produced more female babies, while frozen embryo transfer resulted in more male babies. Thatcher and colleagues [22] reported a higher proportion of male birth after IVF (64%), and Ghazzawi and colleagues [23] reported a higher proportion of female birth after ICSI (61.7%). More recently, Dean et al. [24] retrospectively analyzed the sex of the babies at birth following a single embryo transfer in Australia and New Zealand. There were 13,165 babies born from 13,165 women who had a single embryo transfer (SET) between 2002 and 2006. They reported that ICSI was associated with more females than males and IVF was associated with more males than females. Furthermore, they found that blastocyst transfer was associated with more males than females. They quoted the following sex birth: IVF with a single blastocyst, 56.1% males; IVF with a single cleaved embryo, 51.6 males; ICSI with single blastocyst, 52.5% males; and ICSI with single cleaved embryo, 48.7% males. Recently, Bu et al. [25] analyzed the data of 18 IVF centers in China. There were 62,700 male babies and 58,477 female babies, making the sex ratio 51.8% (male/female = 107:100). In univariate logistic regression analysis, sex ratio was imbalanced toward females at 50.3% when ICSI was performed compared to 47.7% when IVF was used ($P < 0.01$). The sex ratio in IVF/ICSI babies was significantly higher toward males in transfers of blastocyst (54.9%) and thawed embryo (52.4%) than transfers of cleavage stage embryo (51.4%) and fresh embryo (51.5%), respectively. Thus, the IVF technique itself could not change baby sex ratio, while different procedures or methods may change offspring sex ratio [26].

5. Conclusion

Generally speaking, the singleton birth from ART treatment does not have any significant differences from natural conception babies in gestational days, early birth rate, and birthweight, but multiple gestations often resulted in high early birth rate, lower birthweight, and shorter gestational days. The frozen embryo transfer technique may significantly decrease the early birth rate of babies and increase birthweight. Thus, frozen embryo transfer may be recommended as a health strategy in ART. IVF technique itself cannot change sex ratio, but different embryo selection and transfer methods may change sex ratio.

Author details

Linda Wu[1,4], Jinzhou Qin[2,3], Dikai Zhang[2,3,6], Minqi Zhang[2,3], Suzhen Lu[4], Jennifer Howell[5], Timothy J. Gelety[4] and Bin Wu[4]*

1 Department of Physiology, University of Arizona, Tucson, Arizona, USA

2 Department of Reproductive Medicine, The Third Affiliated Hospital of Shenzhen University (Shenzhen Luohu People's Hospital), Shenzhen, Guangdong, China

3 Department of Biology, Southern University of Science and Technology, Shenzhen, Guangdong, China

4 Arizona Center for Reproductive Endocrinology and Infertility, Tucson, AZ, USA

5 Ironwood OB/GYN, A Division of Genesis, Tucson, AZ, USA

6 Department of Gynecology, The Third Affiliated Hospital of Shenzhen University (Shenzhen Luohu People's Hospital), Shenzhen, Guangdong, China

*Address all correspondence to: bwu13@yahoo.com

References

[1] The center for Human Reproduction. PGS no more, long live PGT-A. 2017. Available from: https://www.centerforhumanreprod.com/fertility/pgs-no-long-live-pgt

[2] Niederberger C, Pellicer A. IVF's 40th world birthday. Fertility and Sterility. 2018;**110**(1):4

[3] Bower C, Hansen M. Assisted reproductive technologies and birth outcomes: Overview of recent systematic reviews. Reproduction, Fertility and Development. 2005;**17**:329-333

[4] Fauser BC, Devroey P, Diedrich K, Balaban B, Bonduelle M, Delemarre-van de Waal HA, et al. Health outcomes of children born after IVF/ICSI: A review of current expert opinion and literature. Reproductive Biomedicine Online. 2014;**28**(2):162-182. DOI: 10.1016/j.rbmo.2013.10.013 [Epub Oct 25, 2013]

[5] Klemetti R, Gissle M, Sevon T, Koivurova S, Ritvanen A, Hemminki E. Children born after assisted fertilization have an increased rate of major congenital anomalies. Fertility and Sterility. 2005;**84**(5):1300-1307

[6] Olson CK, Kepple-Noreuil KM, Romitti PA, Budelier WT, Ryan G, Sparks AET, et al. In vitro fertilization is associated with an increase in major birth defects. Fertility and Sterility. 2005;**84**(5):1308-1315

[7] Sutcliffe AG. Congenital anomalies and assisted reproductive technology: More of the same. Fertility and Sterility. 2005;**84**(5):1316-1317

[8] Buckett WM, Tan SL. Congenital abnormalities in children born after assisted reproductive techniques: How much is associated with the presence of infertility and how much with its treatment. Fertility and Sterility. 2005;**84**(5):1318-1319

[9] Schieve LA, Rasmussen SA, Reefhuis J. Risk of birth defects among children conceived with assisted reproductive technology: Providing an epidemiologic context to the data. Fertility and Sterility. 2005;**84**(5):1320-1324

[10] Olivennes F. Do children born after assisted reproductive technology have a higher incidence of birth defects? Fertility and Sterility. 2005;**84**(5):1325-1326

[11] Klemetti R, Gissler M, Sevon T, Koivurova S, Ritcanen A, Hemminki E. Increase evidence of major congenital anomalies in children born with assisted reproductive technology: What should be done? Fertility and Sterility. 2005;**84**(5):1327

[12] Helmerhorst FM, Perquin DAM, Donker D, Kiese MJN. Perinatal outcomes of singletons and twins after assisted conception: A systematic review of controlled studies. British Medical Journal. 2004;**328**:261-265. DOI: 10.1136/BMJ.37957.560278.EE.

[13] Fishel S. First in vitro fertilization baby—This is how it happened. Fertility and Sterility. 2018;**110**(1):5-11

[14] Frydman R. Development of assisted reproductive medicine in Europe. Fertility and Sterility. 2018;**110**(1):12-13

[15] Garcia JE, Rosenwaks Z. Development of in vitro fertilization in the United States: A conversation between Zev Rosenwaks and Jairo E Garcia. Fertility and Sterility. 2018;**110**(1):14-18

[16] Trounson A. Development of in vitro fertilization in Australia. Fertility and Sterility. 2018;**110**(1):19-24

[17] Marcus S. Provides a summary of the complications associated with

IVF pregnancies compared to natural conception. In vitro Fertilization. 2015. http://www.ivf-infertility.com/ivf/standard/outcome.php

[18] Wennerholm U-B, Soderstrom-Anttila V, Bergh C, Aittomaki K, Hazekamp J, Nygren K-G, et al. Children born after cryopreservation of embryos or oocytes: A systematic review of outcome data. Human Reproduction. 2009;**24**(9):2158-2172

[19] Belva F, Henriet S, Van den Abbeel E, Camus M, Devroey P, Van der Elst J, et al. Neonatal outcome of 937 children born after transfer of cryopreserved embryos obtained by ICSI and IVF and comparison with outcome data of fresh ICSI and IVF cycles. Human Reproduction. 2008;**23**(10):2227-2238

[20] Maheshwari A, Pandey S, Raja EA, Shetty A, Hamilton M, Bhattacharya S. Is frozen embryo transfer better for mothers and babies? Can cumulative meta-analysis provide a definitive answer? Human Reproduction Update. 2018;**24**(1):35-58

[21] Wu B. Amplification of Sry gene allows identification of the sex of mouse preimplantation embryos. Theriogenology. 1993;**40**:441-453

[22] Thatcher SS, Restrepo U, Lavy G, DeCherney AH. In-vitro fertilisation and sex ratio. Lancet. 1989;**333**:1025-1026

[23] Ghazzawi IM, Sarraf M, Alhasani S. Children born after ICSI: Are we altering sex ratio? International Journal of Gynecology and Obstetrics. 2000;**70**(Suppl 2):B66

[24] Dean J, Chapman M, Sullivan E. The effect on human sex ratio at birth by assisted reproductive technology (ART) procedures—An assessment of babies born following single embryo transfers, Australia and New Zealand, 2002-2006. BJOG: An International Journal of Obstetrics and Gynaecology. 2010;**117**:1628-1634

[25] Bu Z, Chen Z-J, Huang G, Zhang H, Wu Q, Ma Y, et al. Live birth sex ratio after in vitro fertilization and embryo transfer in china—An analysis of 121,247 babies from 18 centers. PLoS ONE. 2014;**9**(11):e113522. https://doi.org/10.1371/journal.pone.0113522

[26] Pergament E, Todydemir PG, Fiddler M. Sex ratio: A biological perspective of "sex and the city". Reproductive BioMedicine Online. 2002;**5**(1):43-46